System of
Nursing Practice

System of Nursing Practice

A Clinical Nursing Assessment Tool

EILEEN PEARLMAN BECKNELL, R.N., M.N.

Formerly Assistant Professor, College of Nursing
University of Florida, Gainesville

DOROTHY M. SMITH, R.N., M.S.ED.

Dean Emeritus, College of Nursing
University of Florida, Gainesville

F. A. DAVIS COMPANY
PHILADELPHIA

Library of Congress Catalog in Publication Data

Becknell, Eileen Pearlman.
    System of nursing practice.
    Bibliography: p.
    Includes index.
    1. Nurses and nursing. I. Smith, Dorothy Mary, 1913-
joint author. II. Title. [DNLM: 1. Nursing care. WY100 B397s]
RT41.B33   610.73   74-31290
ISBN 0-8036-0695-8

FOREWORD

The need for a systematic approach to the identification and solution of nursing problems has been recognized for at least a quarter of a century. McManus, in 1951, wrote, ". . . the unique function of the professional nurse may be conceived to be: 1) the identification or diagnosis of the nursing problem and the recognition of its interrelated aspects; 2) the deciding upon a course of nursing actions to be followed for the solution of the problem, in light of immediate and long term objectives of nursing, with regard to prevention of illness, direct care, rehabilitation, and promotion of highest standards of health possible for the individual."[1] Such a process requires that the nurse collect information about the patient/client from many sources in a thoughtful, systematic manner in order to have a base upon which to identify nursing problems and determine their solutions.

In the intervening years, nurses have become increasingly aware of the need for accountability in nursing practice, and the need for evaluating the nursing care administered to patients. In addition, the need for systematic recording of the process used in caring for patients as a basis for teaching nursing and for conducting clinical nursing research has become equally evident.

Many people have developed nursing history forms of varying lengths which include varying types and amounts of information. The lack of uniformity in the baseline data necessary for planning nursing care places constraints on the potential for research, evaluation, and teaching clinical nursing practice. As in other professions, standardization of data collection is the keystone for the improvement of nursing practice. It also increases the research potential by furnishing a larger population base to the researcher than one nurse alone can provide.

Other writers have developed texts which describe various parts of the process, such as interviewing, assessment, writing behavioral objectives, decision making, etc. Becknell and Smith, in this book, have included all of the functions essential to planning nursing care using the scientific approach to problem solving. The examples of each part of the process are specifically related to nursing care planning, and are, therefore, very useful since they make the data and the process more meaningful to nursing care. This commends the book to beginning nursing students as well as to practicing nurses.

This text is an initial effort in the development of a standardized approach to the collection of data. It suggests a particular data base and nursing history to be used in planning, implementing, and evaluating nursing care. To the degree that it is successful in leading the profession to a standardized data base, it will have made an important contribution to the nursing profession and to the education of nurses. It will have, in the final analysis, immeasurably advanced the improvement of the quality of nursing care administered to persons in any health care setting.

MARION E. MCKENNA, *Dean of Nursing*
University of Kentucky, Lexington

---

1.   McManus, R. Louise: "Assumptions of functions of nursing," *Regional Planning for Nursing and Nursing Education,* New York, Bureau of Publications, Teachers College, Columbia University, 1951, p. 54.

PREFACE

The development of a scientific nursing practice necessitates the use of the scientific method, that is: 1) the collection of data, 2) the identification of specific problems from the data, 3) the determination of a plan for the solution of each problem, and 4) the evaluation of the progress achieved in solving each problem. The Clinical Nursing Tool developed by Dorothy M. Smith[1] identifies a means of applying the scientific method to nursing, and this text describes the procedure for utilizing this tool in planning and evaluating the nursing care patients receive. It actually describes a process of nursing, discussing thoroughly the specific directions for collecting data, identifying the patient's nursing problems, planning the management of these problems and evaluating the results of the plans. The tool is intended to be used with the Problem-Oriented System which has been described by Weed and others.

It is believed that disciplined, systematic practice of the process described in this book leads to improvement in patient care. While good care is known to exist without a systematic method of nursing practice, it seems to occur by accident, not because it is planned. It is further believed that documentation of this process will, in turn, provide much-needed material for education and clinical research in nursing.[2,3]

This work is written for students and practitioners of baccalaureate nursing programs. In view of the American Nurses' Association's position paper on education for nursing,[4] and believing that the basic skills of the baccalaureate graduate are those involved in the process necessary for the effective use of the Clinical Nursing Tool, the first clinical course in nursing taught by the authors at the University of Florida included this process as "basic skills."[5]

The book is divided into two sections. The first includes those chapters pertaining to background information and purposes of the tool, and the collection, organization, and recording of data (Part A of the Clinical Nursing Tool). The second section consists of those chapters pertaining to the process of clinical thinking, that is, identifying patients' nursing problems, developing a plan of care, and evaluating the results of the plan (Part B of the Clinical Nursing Tool).

EILEEN PEARLMAN BECKNELL
DOROTHY M. SMITH

1. Smith, Dorothy M.: "A clinical nursing tool," *American Journal of Nursing.* 68:2384–2388, 1968.
2. Ibid.
3. Smith, Dorothy M.: "Myth and method in nursing practice," *American Journal of Nursing.* 64:68–72, 1964.
4. "American Nurses' Association's First Position on Education for Nursing," *American Journal of Nursing.* 65:106–111, 1965.
5. Smith, Dorothy M.: "A clinical nursing tool," *American Journal of Nursing.* 68:2388, 1968.

ACKNOWLEDGMENTS

We would like to acknowledge the contribution of Dr. Marion E. McKenna who wrote a preliminary manual which preceded the work included in this text. Collaboration with Dr. McKenna helped us to write some of the material included here.

We would especially like to acknowledge and thank the many patients who gave us valuable data and the opportunity to practice the process described in this text. Without their help and the opportunity to practice, we would not have been able to identify and make the revisions we found necessary as we worked with the process. We thank them for helping us to learn.

Finally, we would like to recognize the contribution of the faculty and students of the University of Florida College of Nursing. Their questions and comments helped us to clarify our thinking and, in turn, the material included in this book.

CONTENTS

SECTION ONE

Background

1

INTRODUCTION

This chapter is designed to give the reader an understanding of the frame of reference in which this text is written. The development and clinical application of the system are briefly explained in five parts: 1) definitions of particular terms used throughout the text, 2) rationale for the development of the Clinical Nursing Tool, 3) purposes of the Clinical Nursing Tool, 4) particular data collection guide chosen (the Nursing History), and 5) organization of the data collection guide.

DEFINITIONS

As a basis for understanding the material contained in this work, the following terms are defined:

Clinical Nursing Tool—an instrument developed by Dorothy M. Smith at the University of Florida College of Nursing to serve ". . . as a guide in eliciting and organizing certain data that might be used to plan nursing care, to describe research problems, to teach students, to develop standards, and to evaluate care."[1] Furthermore, it outlines a process of clinical thinking, based on the obtained data, which is advocated for solving problems in nursing care. (See Appendix 1.)

Nursing History—the written systematic organization of patient data collected according to the guide outlined in Part A of the Clinical Nursing Tool. (See Appendix 1.)

Scientific Method—a procedure for approaching a question, situation, person, or idea according to a definitely established, logical and systematic plan. (See Appendix 2.)

Process—a systematic series of actions directed toward achieving a definite result. In this instance, the series of steps the nurse takes in planning and evaluating nursing care, using the process of clinical thinking outlined in Part B of the Clinical Nursing Tool. (See Appendix 1.)

Problem—any question proposed for solution or consideration; anything

3

required to be done. As used in this text, a problem is any condition or situation in which a patient requires help to maintain or regain a state of health, or to achieve a peaceful death. A problem may concern the patient, the patient's family and/or the nurse.

Problem-Oriented System—a system, developed by Dr. Lawrence L. Weed,[2] for recording information in the patient's chart. The system is designed for use in improving the quality of patient care and to provide data which may be utilized for medical education and research. In this case, it provides data to be used in nursing practice, education, and research. This work has been prepared for use with this system.

THE NEED FOR A SYSTEM

Smith has written about the lack of a system of nursing practice, rather than the lack of motivation, education, or knowledge, as being the cause of inadequate nursing care.[3,4] She states that we need ". . . an organized framework wherein we can see plainly and definitely what is to be done and what we must do to accomplish it."[5] In an article in 1964, she asked several pertinent questions:

What system do we presently have for insuring good nursing care? What procedure that makes it mandatory for the team leader to know as much about each individual patient as is necessary to insure his best care? What method for assessing patients' nursing problems and for dealing with them—and for evaluating both assessment and management?[6]

Furthermore, Smith states that ". . . a system, in and of itself, does not guarantee that the care that is given will be adequate. But . . . without a system, without some plan of operation, adequate care will never be given, except by chance or by accident."[7]

The system of practice discussed above is now often referred to as the *nursing process*. Regardless of the specific steps outlined, it is generally accepted that the nursing process involves the ability to make an assessment, identify nursing care problems based on patient needs, decide how to deal with or solve these problems, and then evaluate whether the prescribed methods did indeed effect a satisfactory resolution. Although usage of the term nursing process is widespread and general information about it is abundant, specific information and examples demonstrating each step are scarce. Therefore, students and practitioners are left to guess at a method of practice and never know whether they are meeting the "standard" which has not been stated.

In 1968, Smith[3] described the search for and development of a procedure to make the functions involved in the nursing process operational. The result was the Clinical Nursing Tool. Except for minor revisions, this is the tool for which this text is written.

4

PURPOSES OF CLINICAL NURSING TOOL

While providing a means of systematically organizing data, the Clinical Nursing Tool has several other purposes:

1. The clinical tool provides the means for individualized nursing care based upon the patient's patterns, preferences and problems, as well as scientific knowledge.

2. The use of the clinical tool assists the nurse in setting priorities. It is impossible to meet all of a person's needs. By formulating a problem list, the nurse identifies all the needs which she feels require nursing attention. She then selects those problems which are of most immediate concern, and these take priority over others presented by the patient. Therefore, problems are not just "accidentally taken care of," but are deliberately and systematically solved.

3. The nursing history, problem list, plan of care, and progress notes provide a record for evaluating the quality of nursing care. Both nursing objectives and patient response to nursing care are recorded in patient behavioral terms. Thus, progress toward achievement of these objectives can be evaluated and current methods modified if necessary. Without a written record which may be analyzed in terms of whether the patient's nursing problems were solved, evaluation of nursing care is an amorphous procedure based on individual value judgments rather than scientific criteria.

4. The tool provides consistent, systematic collection of data for use in setting standards. If nursing care is to have a quality of "good" or "poor," it must be measured against constants—good in relation to what? or poor in terms of what standard? Abdellah[8] states that measurable criteria have not been established for effective patient care. She feels that this is due, in part, to the fact that nursing has not identified a body of knowledge against which nursing practice can be correlated. Valid and reliable criteria that are also measurable are needed to evaluate and promote patient progress.

Uniform collection of data makes it possible to define commonalities in nursing problems, methods for solving the problems, and the successes or failures of these methods. If given a sufficient quantity of data, it then becomes possible to predict outcomes of nursing approaches to particular situations. The final result is that the quality of care may then be determined by the predicted outcomes with any given set of problems and approaches, and the evaluation of care may be based on data, rather than on the values of the individuals performing the evaluation.

Standards in nursing also promote a greater degree of efficiency by reducing the trial and error approach to the solution of nursing problems. This, in turn, reduces the frustrations of nursing personnel and increases job satisfaction by providing more accuracy in prescribing nursing measures, predicting outcomes, and evaluating results.

5. The nursing history, problem list, plan of care, and progress notes

provide a system for consistent communication of patient information to all personnel involved. This lessens the problems of verbal reports at shift changes of personnel, and also aids when patients are transferred from one unit to another or when they are discharged to another agency.

6. Systematic use of the tool provides a descriptive record for teaching nursing students the scientific method of problem solving. The role of the professional nurse dictates that the student learn to assume responsibility for making the necessary assessment and develop the nursing methods to assist the patient. This is a skill which is acquired by practice using a consistent pattern of data collection, planning, and evaluation as supplied by the clinical tool. The student sees the data which have been collected and utilized by practicing nurses and thus learns the thinking process involved in assessing, planning, and evaluating nursing care.

7. Finally, the clinical tool provides a means whereby areas for nursing research may be more clearly defined. Nurses will be able to identify recurring nursing problems, relationships between pieces of data, and successful nursing methods. This knowledge will guide the planning of research projects and thus further the development of a scientific nursing process.

SELECTION OF DATA COLLECTION GUIDE

The development of a scientific nursing practice necessitates the use of the scientific method. The first two steps of this process are collection of data, and identification of specific problems from that data. This raises two basic questions: 1) What data must nurses collect from patients? and 2) What problems are nurses required to assess and manage? Before answering these questions, it is necessary to define the term *nursing*. We have used Henderson's definition:

Nursing is primarily assisting the individual, sick or well, in the performance of those activities contributing to health or its recovery (or to a peaceful death) that he would perform unaided if he had the necessary strength, will, or knowledge. It is likewise the unique contribution of nursing to help the individual to be independent of such assistance as soon as possible.[9]

According to Henderson, ". . . the nurse is the authority on basic nursing care."[10] She defines basic nursing care as helping the patient with the following activities or providing the conditions under which he can perform them unaided:

1. Breathe normally.
2. Eat and drink adequately.
3. Eliminate body wastes.

6

4. Move and maintain desirable postures.
5. Sleep and rest.
6. Select suitable clothes—dress and undress.
7. Maintain body temperature within normal range by adjusting clothing and modifying the environment.
8. Keep the body clean and well groomed and protect the integument.
9. Avoid dangers in the environment and avoid injuring others.
10. Communicate with others expressing emotions, needs, fears, or opinions.
11. Worship according to one's faith.
12. Work in such a way that there is a sense of accomplishment.
13. Play or participate in various forms of recreation.
14. Learn, discover, or satisfy the curiosity that leads to normal development and health and use the available health facilities.[11]

Thus, it can be seen that nursing assists the individual toward health—both mental and physical. The term assists implies that the patient is an active participant in his care and that the nurse helps him by utilizing *his* strengths and coping patterns whenever possible.

There are several assumptions which further serve as a frame of reference for the development and use of the Nursing History:

1. There are life-supporting activities (adaptive processes or patterns). These include those activities identified above by Henderson.
2. There are differences in how these patterns are maintained.
3. Most people have opinions as to how to best maintain these activities even though standards have been developed through research and/or usage. Some of these opinions are consistent with the standards and some are not.
4. The person is the best source of information concerning his life-supporting activities and their maintenance.
5. There are times in the lives of all persons when help is needed in the maintenance of some or all of these life-supporting processes.

Now the question, "What data must nurses collect from patients?" can begin to be answered. The nurse should collect data concerning the patient's life-supporting activities, his individual patterns of maintaining them, and any difficulties involved. Using this data, she can then determine the best method of assistance.

Abdellah and her associates identify 21 groups of common nursing problems which resulted from two studies by the Division of Nursing Resources of the United States Public Health Service from 1953 to 1955 and a third study in cooperation with the National League for Nursing from 1955 to 1958.[12] This list identifies the areas which nurses are called upon to assess and manage.

1. Maintain good hygiene and physical comfort.
2. Promote optimal activity: exercise, rest, and sleep.
3. Promote safety through prevention of accident, injury, or other trauma and through the prevention of the spread of infection.
4. Maintain good body mechanics and prevent and correct deformities.
5. Facilitate the maintenance of a supply of oxygen to all body cells.
6. Facilitate the maintenance of nutrition of all body cells.
7. Facilitate the maintenance of elimination.
8. Facilitate the maintenance of fluid and electrolyte balance.
9. Recognize the physiologic responses of the body to disease conditions—pathologic, physiologic, and compensatory.
10. Facilitate the maintenance of regulatory mechanisms and functions.
11. Facilitate the maintenance of sensory function.
12. Identify and accept positive and negative expressions, feelings, and reactions.
13. Identify and accept the interrelatedness of emotions and organic illness.
14. Facilitate the maintenance of effective verbal and nonverbal communication.
15. Promote the development of productive interpersonal relationships.
16. Facilitate progress toward achievement of personal spiritual goals.
17. Create and/or maintain a therapeutic environment.
18. Facilitate awareness of self as an individual with varying physical, emotional, and developmental needs.
19. Accept the optimum possible goals in the light of limitations, physical and emotional.
20. Use community resources as an aid in resolving problems arising from illness.
21. Understand the role of social problems as influencing factors in the cause of illness.

In summary, the data which the nurse must collect from patients is that pertaining to the life-supporting activities. The 21 items above outline the categories of problems or areas which the nurse must assess and manage. The actual specific statement of the problem can only occur after careful collection of data and study of the individual patient.

ORGANIZATION OF THE NURSING HISTORY

The rationale for the present structure of the Nursing History is included here to assist in better understanding its organization. (See Part A of Appendix 1.)

Much of the data for the first category, "Vital Statistics," can be obtained from the patient's addressograph or chart. This gives the nurse factual, objective information before she meets the patient, which may make her feel more comfortable. Using this information, such as calling the patient by name or indicating that she knows where the patient lives, may make the patient feel more at ease. In this way the patient is also informed that there is a source of information about him for use by health personnel, and that members of the staff are communicating.

The second category, "Patient's Understanding of Illness," is the first major category about which the patient is required to give information. Because the patient usually wants to talk about his troubles and why he came to the hospital,[13] the beginning establishment of the nurse-patient relationship can take place through the discussion of this category. When the patient is encouraged to talk about what is of major concern to him, he becomes more willing to give information in later categories. In addition to ascertaining the patient's perception of his condition, the data included in this category alert the nurse to the patient's most immediate needs and nursing problems.

The third category, "Some Indications of the Patient's Expectations," serves much the same purpose as the second category. Understanding the patient's expectations helps the nurse to understand his behavior while indicating to the patient that the nurse is interested in finding ways to make his stay in the hospital more comfortable.

The data in the fourth category, "Brief Social and Cultural History," give the nurse an indication of those persons and events which affect the patient and his behavior.

The information included in the first four categories can be used as a guide for questions the nurse asks in the fifth category, "Significant Data in Terms of . . . ," and the sixth category, "That Which Makes the Patient Feel Cared For."

The fifth category provides information pertaining to the patient's usual patterns of living (his life-supporting activities). This information helps the nurse determine what, if any, problems the patient is experiencing and what he has found to be effective in helping him cope. This data provides a baseline from which to begin a plan of care and measure change. While the patient's usual patterns of living can never be replicated in the hospital, the plan of care can be made to incorporate some of these patterns. It must be remembered that it is not possible to meet all of the patient's needs either in the hospital or out; however, the nurse will find that the patient's fears and anxieties associated with illness and hospitalization are most effectively allayed through such reassurances as may be offered by the familiar routines to which he is accustomed.

The data in the sixth category help the nurse determine those things which contribute to the patient's comfort and feeling of being cared for. This feeling may derive from: familiar routines and environmental circumstances, the possession of material objects, or religious beliefs and practices. The positive attitudes and actions of significant others toward

9

these feelings tell the individual that he is worthy of attention, assistance or concern, and thus provide the reassurance necessary for health.

These last two categories were arranged with Maslow's hierarchy of needs in mind. (Since the tool was first developed, the subcategories K and L have been added; thus, the organization in terms of Maslow's hierarchy of needs is not complete.) It is felt that an understanding of Maslow's theory of needs and needs hierarchy will aid in understanding the data collected in the Nursing History, its organization, and application.

MASLOW'S HIERARCHY OF NEEDS[14]

A *need* may be defined as a condition requiring supply or relief; the lack of something requisite, desired, wanted, useful, or deemed necessary.[15] According to Maslow, there are five categories of basic needs:

1. Physiologic needs
2. Safety needs
3. Love and belongingness needs
4. Esteem needs, and
5. Self-actualization needs.

These basic needs are interrelated and arranged in a hierarchy of dominance. The most dominant need will monopolize consciousness and organize the various capacities of the person, while the less dominant needs are minimized or even forgotten. However, when a need is fairly well satisfied, the next dominant or higher need emerges and serves as the center of organization of behavior.

Physiologic Needs. The physiologic needs are the most basic and most dominant of all needs. They are those necessary for survival and include breathing, eating, drinking, activity, and so on. The first six subcategories of the fifth category in the Nursing History are primarily concerned with physiologic needs. These must be at least minimally gratified for the individual to be concerned with his other (higher) needs.

Safety Needs. If the physiologic needs are relatively well gratified, there emerges a new set of needs which are categorized as safety needs. The average person in our society prefers a safe, orderly, predictable, organized world, in which unexpected, unmanageable, or dangerous things do not occur. This can be seen in the preference for undisrupted routine, a predictable schedule, and the need for consistency. Confronting the average individual with new, unfamiliar, or unmanageable stimuli or situations will frequently elicit a danger or terror reaction. Therefore, the attempt to seek safety and stability is seen in the common preference for the known rather than the unknown.

Love and Belongingness Needs. When both the physiologic and safety needs are gratified, the love, affection and belongingness needs emerge as

10

the focus of the individual and his behavior. The love needs involve both giving and receiving. The person will seek affectionate relationships with people, a place in his group, and will feel strongly the absence of family and friends. Gratification of these needs enables one to express warmth, kindness, and consideration toward others.

Esteem Needs. All people have a need or desire for a stable, high evaluation of themselves and for the respect of others. This is manifested in the desire for strength, achievement, confidence, independence, prestige, and appreciation by others. Satisfaction of these needs leads to feelings of selfconfidence, worth, strength and capability, while thwarting them produces feelings of inferiority, weakness, and helplessness.

Self-Actualization Needs. Even if the physiologic, safety, love, and esteem needs are satisfied, a new discontent may soon develop unless the individual is fulfilling his capabilities. This is called the need for self-actualization. This category of needs includes the need for self-identity, self-realization, self-direction, and self-fulfillment. The specific manner in which these needs are manifested varies greatly.

While the physiologic needs can be discussed directly, it is more difficult to discuss safety, love and belongingness, or esteem needs in a direct manner since most people do not know or are unable to say how they meet these needs. All human behavior is purposeful and seeks to fulfill some need. Any interference with the satisfaction of a need leads to frustration, and repeated frustration causes anxiety.[16] This resulting anxiety may lead to many different kinds of behavior which can only be understood on an individual basis. The categories of "Interpersonal and Communicative Patterns," "Temperament," "Dependency and Independency Patterns," and "That which helps the patient feel safe, secure, comfortable, protected, and cared for," sometimes produce clues to how the patient sees his psychologic needs being met and gives the nurse an indication of his usual coping behavior when they are not.

SATISFACTION OF NEEDS

The most basic consequence of satisfying any need is that this need is submerged and a higher need emerges.[17] Therefore, the appearance of a need depends upon the previous satisfaction of a more basic one. For example, a person who has had none of his basic needs satisfied will most likely be motivated by the physiologic needs rather than any others. In other words, ". . . a person who is lacking food, safety, love, and esteem would most probably hunger for food more strongly than for anything else."[18] As Peplau says, "All behavior aims to reduce tension arising from needs. When a strong need is uppermost, all behavior is directed toward it and other needs may be unrecognized."[19]

Peplau also states that, "When immediate needs are met more mature needs arise."[20] This is shown by the pattern of progress up the hierarchy:

11

need—satisfaction, higher need—satisfaction, still higher need—satisfaction. Therefore, nurses must assist patients to meet their present needs, thus enabling more mature needs to dominate. Needs which are consistently gratified cease to function as active determinants of behavior. They now exist only in a potential fashion, in that they may emerge again to dominate the person if they are thwarted. ". . . a want that is satisfied is no longer a want."[21]

Through gratification, people develop the ability to withstand thwarting of needs and to delay satisfaction, called "increased frustration tolerance through early gratification."[22] Therefore, individuals in whom a certain need has generally been satisfied can better tolerate deprivation than those who have been consistently deprived.

This hierarchy of basic needs is not completely rigid. Although most people have basic needs which appear in the sequence presented, any of these needs may become dominant at any time without following the given order.

SUMMARY

This chapter presents the operational frame of reference. While we cannot make explicit all our values, it should be stated that there are two assumptions that have been very important in guiding our work:

1. Primary relationships between nurses and patients are a significant factor in the healing process.
2. Prevalent nursing service organizational structures and prevalent curricula and teaching methods in schools of nursing do not provide systematic, sustained, and supervised opportunities for such primary relationships.

Health agencies have responded to changes such as health insurance, shortages of professional and skilled health personnel, growth of auxiliary health fields, and major advances in medicine and drug therapy, but have done little to meet the needs of patients internally—to modify their own operational structures and functions so that the patient feels he is something more than an immobilized sick person. Outside the confines of the family, there is no more exposed or intimate environment in which a person finds himself. Emotionally and socially, however, he is typically neglected, finding the usual hospital situation anxiety producing due to lack of the usual reinforcements of his social contacts. Basic integrative and supportive elements in the life patterns of any individual are found in interactions with others—primary type relationships. Therefore, establishing primary type relationships should be an integral part of the nursing process. However, Menzies shows that nursing services are organized in such a way as to deliberately set up distance between the nurse and the patient as a defense against anxiety.[23] This attitude discourages the establishment of necessary relationships both between nurse and patient and among members of the health team. The system of nursing practice described in this text fosters primary type relationships and the use of cognitive skills as a more satisfactory defense against anxiety.

REFERENCES

1. Smith, Dorothy M.: "A clinical nursing tool." *American Journal of Nursing* 68:2387, 1968.
2. Weed, Lawrence L.; *Medical Records, Medical Education and Patient Care.* The Press of Case Western Reserve University, Cleveland, Year Book Medical Publishers, Inc., Chicago, 1969.
3. Smith, op. cit., pp. 2384–2388.
4. Smith, Dorothy M.: "Myth and method in nursing practice." *American Journal of Nursing* 64:68–72, 1964.
5. Ibid., p. 68.
6. Ibid., p. 71.
7. Ibid., p. 69.
8. Abdellah, Faye G.: "Criterion measures in nursing." *Nursing Research,* 10:21–26, 1961.
9. Harmer, Bertha, and Henderson, Virginia: *Textbook of the Principles and Practice of Nursing,* fifth edition. The Macmillan Company, New York, 1957, p. 4.
10. Henderson, Virginia: *The Nature of Nursing: A Definition and Its Implications for Practice, Research and Education.* The Macmillan Company, New York, 1966, p. 16.
11. Ibid., pp. 16, 17.
12. Abdellah, Faye G., et al.: *Patient Centered Approaches to Nursing.* The Macmillan Company, New York, 1964, pp. 12–17.
13. Herrmann, George R.: *Clinical Case-Taking,* fourth edition. The C. V. Mosby Company, St. Louis, 1949, pp. 25–27.
14. Maslow, Abraham H.: "A theory of human motivation." *Psychological Review* 50:370–396, 1943.
15. *Webster's New Collegiate Dictionary.* G. and C. Merriam Company, Publishers, Springfield, 1960, p. 562.
16. Peplau, Hildegard E.: *Interpersonal Relations in Nursing.* G. P. Putnam's Sons, New York, 1952, pp. 86–93.
17. Maslow, Abraham H.: *Motivation and Personality.* Harper and Row, Publishers, New York, 1954, p. 108.
18. Maslow, Abraham H.: "A theory of human motivation." *Psychological Review* 50:373, 1943.
19. Peplau, op. cit., p. 80.
20. Ibid., p. 79.
21. Maslow, Abraham H.: "A theory of human motivation." *Psychological Review* 50:375, 1943.
22. Ibid., p. 387.
23. Menzies, Isabel E. P.: *The Functioning of Social Systems as a Defense Against Anxiety.* Centre for Applied Social Research, The Tavistock Institute of Human Relations, Tavistock Centre, London, 1970.

2

THE PROBLEM-ORIENTED SYSTEM

The problem-oriented system developed by Weed is a method of organizing and recording information in the patient's chart and provides a systematic method for planning and evaluating patient care.[1] This system can be used to apply the scientific method of problem solving to the management of nursing care. It is a logical progression involving the following five phases:[2]

1. *The Data Base.* On admission or as soon as possible thereafter, patient information is collected (the Nursing History) which serves as the basis for planning nursing care.

2. *The Problem List.* Following the initial collection of data, a numbered list of problems is formulated, including problems identified from the Nursing History and from information recorded by other members of the health team. New problems are added to the list as they are identified. The list serves as a table of contents for the patient's chart (if all members of the health team use the same problem list) or to the record of nursing care (if nursing notes are separated from physician's notes).

3. *The Initial Plan.* A plan is prepared for the solution of each problem on the list. The plan consists of one or more of the following: 1) collection of additional pertinent data, 2) transmission of information to patient or others, and 3) statement of nursing care objectives and orders designed to solve or manage the specified problem.

4. *The Progress Notes.* This phase is comprised of the chronological sequence of notes pertaining to the evaluation of progress in the management of each problem, additional data, new plans, and modification or deletion of old plans.

5. *The Discharge or Transfer Note.* This final phase of the problem-oriented system is a summary of the patient's nursing problems, noting those which were resolved and recommendations for the management of those still present. In this sense, the discharge or transfer note represents a final progress note.

THE SCIENTIFIC METHOD

The following explanation demonstrates more specifically how the stages of the scientific method are applied through each phase of the problem-oriented system. (See Appendix 2.)

1. *Collection of Data.* This is provided by the Nursing History, the first phase of the problem-oriented system.

2. *Identification of Specific Problems from the Data.* The problem list, the second phase of the problem-oriented system, serves this purpose.

3. *Statement of Specific Plans for the Solution of Each Problem.* Useful, realistic, and scientifically sound plans must be based upon the study of existing knowledge and factors related to the problem. This necessitates the collection, description, and classification of relevant data by direct observation and/or from the literature. This is termed the *inductive stage of inquiry.* One must then consider relevant hypotheses and formulate postulates (assumptions) from each major hypothesis. It is these postulates which become evident in the nursing care objectives and subsequent nursing orders written to achieve them. In essence, the orders say, "If these activities are performed, the goal will be achieved." This is the third phase of the problem-oriented system.

4. *Record of Continuing Evaluation of Progress Achieved in Solving Each Problem.* This record is the fourth stage of the problem-oriented system, the progress notes. In this testing stage, hypotheses are verified or refuted. This is referred to as the *deductive stage of inquiry.* The progress notes reflect whether or not the plan of care is solving the original problem, and thus whether a hypothesis and its postulates are correct or incorrect. If objectives are not being achieved the nurse must choose another hypothesis or modify her plan of care, and the testing and evaluating are repeated. When certain hypotheses repeatedly yield the same results, generalizations may be made for use in similar situations.

It is these four stages which are evident in the written record. It must be recognized, however, that while each stage of the scientific method is not documented in the record, it is essential that the nurse's thinking proceed through each of these stages in a systematic manner. For example, the nurse must consider what is already known about a problem and its methods of solution in order to write scientifically sound plans even though she does not record in the chart everything she finds through her search of the literature.

USE OF THE PROBLEM-ORIENTED SYSTEM

Weed refers to the problem-oriented system as a "tool." He says that "a tool facilitates, and in some cases for the first time makes possible progress toward a goal; it guarantees nothing."[3] When properly used, the tool allows the nurse to progress in her attempt to define the patient's nursing

16

problems, organize plans for their management, and evaluate the quality of nursing care actually given.

The progression toward these goals cannot be achieved unless there are rules established to guide the nurse. Hurst states, "Excellence in sports, art, science, or medicine cannot be pursued, achieved, or measured without appropriate rules."[4] Therefore, if the advantages of the system are to be realized, adherence to the rules is necessary. Errors made in performing just one aspect of the system may affect the remainder, and thus the management of a patient's nursing care. According to Randall, ". . . even simple errors can make the system seem cumbersome and difficult to use."[5] Explanations of the rules pertaining to each phase of the system are included in later chapters.

Strict adherence to the guidelines established by Weed does not limit thought and creativity. They are simply the framework within which excellence can be pursued, achieved, and measured. The system allows the nurse freedom to make independent judgments about *nursing* problems and their management within a definite framework to guide and support the decision-making process.[6] Hurst states:

When there are no rules pertaining to the records, the performance of a physician cannot be judged. The physician cannot even judge himself. He cannot define his problems. He cannot improve because there are no identifiable, reproducible obstacles to work against.[7]

The above statement is just as accurate if the word nurse is substituted for the word physician.

SUMMARY

The problem-oriented system is a tool through which the scientific method of problem solving can be applied to the management of nursing care. Using the Clinical Nursing Tool in conjunction with this system furthers progress toward goals in planning individualized care, evaluating its quality, developing standards, obtaining data for teaching purposes, and defining areas for clinical nursing research. Only in this manner can we achieve our ultimate aim of improved nursing care.

REFERENCES

1. Weed, Lawrence L.: *Medical Records, Medical Education and Patient Care*. The Press of Case Western Reserve University, Cleveland, Year Book Medical Publishers, Inc., Chicago, 1969.
2. Ibid., p. 13.
3. Weed, Lawrence L.: "Questions often asked about the problem-oriented record— Does it guarantee quality?" in Hurst, J., and Walker, H. K. (eds.): *The Problem-Oriented System*. MEDCOM, Inc., New York, 1972, p. 51.

4. Hurst, J. Willis: "The problem-oriented record and the measurement of excellence." *Archives of Internal Medicine* 128:819, 1971.
5. Randall, R. Beauvais: "Errors frequently made in using the problem-oriented system," in Hurst, J., and Walker, H. K. (eds.): *The Problem-Oriented System*. MED-COM, Inc., New York, 1972, p. 67.
6. Bloom, Judith T., et al.: "Problem-oriented charting." *American Journal of Nursing* 71:2146, 1971.
7. Hurst, op. cit.

3

BASELINE DATA

The first part of this chapter is a discussion of baseline data, its definition, rationale, and the development of the particular data base used in this
text. The chapter then proceeds to outline baseline data included within the
categories of the Nursing History, discuss recording of the written history,
and provide an example of a Nursing History.

The word data denotes facts or information.[1] A base is the foundation,
groundwork, or support; that from which a commencement or start is
made.[2] Therefore, the terms *baseline data* and *data base* as used in this text
are defined as *information derived from the patient which serves as a
starting point for planning nursing care.*

The baseline data is intended to be the minimum information recorded in
a patient's Nursing History. Its purpose is to provide enough information
to identify significant nursing problems, not to gather all possible data
about a problem and its solution. However, this is not meant to inhibit the
individual nurse from recording additional information as determined by
her knowledge, experience, and observations during the interview.

Based on her knowledge pertaining to specific groups of patients (such as
maternity patients or surgical patients), specific disease conditions (such as
diabetes or arthritis), and normal physiologic and psychologic functions,
the nurse may collect certain data from a particular patient which she
would not collect in all cases. It is the nurse's decision whether she gathers
only the baseline data during the Nursing History or whether she attempts
to collect additional data at this time or during later interactions with the
patient. Experience has shown that the baseline data provide the information necessary to begin a plan of care and that additional data are best
collected after the nurse has had the opportunity to consider what other
specific information she requires and how to gather it. However, many
patients volunteer valuable information which the nurse does not actively
elicit as part of the data base, but which may be recorded in the Nursing
History.

19

The problem-oriented system advocated by Weed requires that the data base be defined. A *defined data base* is one in which the content, or data to be collected, has been previously stated. There is no such thing as a "complete" Nursing History. However, if the information to be collected is determined in advance, it is possible to obtain the same data from every patient and thus obtain a complete Nursing History in terms of the established standard. Weed compares defining the data base with establishing the rules for a football game:

Failure to define the initial data base is like playing football with a different number of men each time on a field of no definite length. Individual plays can be perfected, but their value is unclear because their context is not constant and complete.[3]

He further states that:

Once the desirable data base has been defined, individual modifications in it should not be allowed, even as rationalizations proceeding from limitations on staff time or other troublesome professional circumstances. Uniformity in data base is among the important factors tending to permit accurate comparability and generalization, and it is essential to the welfare of the whole patient. Both for the sake of our science and the sake of our patient, the standard data base must conscientiously be sought on each patient. . . .[4]

The defined data base serves to obtain necessary information and exclude irrelevant material. Bjorn and Cross state:

Once this data base is established, the task of determining the data base for each individual patient no longer exists, and time can be devoted to collecting the information rather than to wondering what information to collect.[5]

Members of the medical profession do not agree on any particular defined data base.[6] Therefore, it is hardly surprising that nursing has a multitude of different data collection guides and disagreement about what should constitute the baseline data collected on every patient. Weed states that complete agreement in this area is not necessary; the data base should merely conform to the following rules:

1. Is defined, explicit, and thorough enough to at least start action on problems you feel you cannot afford to miss.
2. Is obtained every time.
3. Is reliable.[7]

The data base defined in this chapter evolved over a period of years. The first list of data to be included in a Nursing History was developed as a guide to give beginning nursing students an idea of the data they needed to obtain. Since this method required collecting as much data as possible pertaining to each category, the amount of time and patience involved on the part of both nurse and patient proved prohibitive. Subsequent revisions were based on the following questions:

1. What data seem to apply to the majority of patients rather than to the exceptions?
2. What data are helpful in planning nursing care that are not already included elsewhere in a patient's chart?
3. What is the least amount of data pertaining to the majority of patients that is needed:
   a. To learn something about the patient as a person,
   b. To identify the patient's usual patterns within the categories of the Nursing History, and
   c. To identify problems the patient may have related to the categories of the Nursing History?

Bjorn and Cross state that although the data base must have flexibility to change as a result of evaluation or new information, "when undue flexibility is permitted from patient to patient, however, chaos results. . . ."[8] Having defined the data base, it should now be used for a large number of patients over a significant period of time and then evaluated for possible modification. This provides for elimination of data which are nonproductive and/or addition of data which are consistently needed initially, yet not required in the current data base.

The feasibility of acquiring a "complete" Nursing History on every patient has been questioned. While there are exceptions, experience with this tool has shown that it is possible to obtain a thorough history from the majority of patients. Depending upon individual circumstances, the collection process may require days, weeks, or even months. For example, if a newly admitted patient is experiencing pain, the nurse may be able to collect some data but most likely would not attempt to obtain the entire Nursing History. Therefore, as Problem #1 on the problem list, she would write "incomplete data base" and indicate her plans for completion of the data collection.[9] This is discussed further in Chapters 6 and 7.

The following outline defines the baseline data to be recorded in the Nursing History. This includes those items which have been found helpful in planning the initial nursing care for a majority of patients. Information primarily concerned with the patient's usual (prehospitalization) patterns within these categories is used to maintain these coping mechanisms, as far as possible, while the patient is in the hospital.

BASELINE DATA INCLUDED IN THE NURSING HISTORY

I. Vital Statistics
   A. Name
   B. Age
   C. Sex
   D. Marital status
   E. City of residence
   F. Number of hospital admissions

II. Patient's Understanding of Illness
   A. State what happened to make the patient come to the hospital at this time.
      (*Note:* If the patient uses a technical term, such as diabetes, seizures, spells, depressed, heart attack, and so on, clarify and record specifically what he experiences.)
   B. Describe the events in the patient's life (in his family, work, and/or social relationships) about the time he began noticing any indication of illness. In addition, note:
      1. Time of onset
      2. Who he was with
      3. What he was doing.
   C. Describe the effect this illness has had on the patient's habits of living.

III. Some Indications of the Patient's Expectations
   A. Describe what the patient expects to occur during this hospitalization.
   B. Describe what the patient expects as a result of this hospitalization.
   C. Describe the patient's expectations regarding his nursing care.
      (*Note:* This is not intended to be a request for an evaluation of past or present nursing care or nurses. If the patient begins an evaluation, interrupt him and tell him that you are not asking him for an evaluation. This item is concerned with what the patient wants or would like. Most patients are able to give this information once they know that they are not being asked to evaluate nurses and/or nursing care.)

IV. Brief Social and Cultural History
   A. Occupation; if retired, state former occupation.
   B. Educational background (level achieved).
      (*Note:* If below fourth grade, determine the patient's ability to read and write.)
   C. List the members of the patient's immediate family. In addition, record:
      1. Who he lives with or that he lives alone.

D. State the person (persons) who is (are) most significant, important to this patient. If the patient cannot identify a person, consider:
　　1. Animals, things
　　2. Church, work, organizations, and so on.
E. Describe anything about which the patient is concerned or worried at this time (family, work, finances, and so on).
V. Significant Data in Terms of
　A. Sleeping patterns
　　1. State usual bedtime; time wakes up. (Include the time patient gets up if different from when he wakes up.)
　　2. Describe bedtime rituals (such as, eating, drinking, bathing, reading, smoking, and so on). Include:
　　　a. Rituals in preparing for sleep
　　　b. Rituals which the patient perceives as helping him to sleep.
　　3. Describe problems the patient experiences related to falling asleep or waking up during the night.
　　　a. If the patient has difficulty falling asleep, either initially or after having been asleep, note:
　　　　(1) Those measures he employs to help him sleep
　　　　(2) The activity in which he engages while awake
　　　　(3) That which he thinks about while awake.
　　　b. If the patient wakes up during the night, note:
　　　　(1) Why he wakes up
　　　　(2) The number of times he wakes up
　　　　(3) Any problems he has going back to sleep.
　　4. Note the number of pillows used by the patient.
　B. Eliminating patterns
　　1. State the usual frequency of bowel movements. In addition, note:
　　　a. The date of the patient's last bowel movement.
　　2. Record that which the patient perceives as contributing to the maintenance of his pattern. Include what is used and when. (Aids may include coffee, juices, eating, activity, laxatives, and so on.)
　　3. Describe any difficulty the patient experiences with bowel elimination, i.e., pain, diarrhea, constipation, and so on. (*Note:* The interviewer must determine and record what the patient means by "constipation," "diarrhea," "difficulty," and so on.)
　　4. If the patient does experience any difficulty describe what he does to prevent and/or alleviate the difficulty.
　　5. Describe any difficulty the patient experiences with voiding, i.e., frequency, pain, burning, bleeding, and so on. (*Note:* The interviewer must clarify and record what the patient means by frequency, how often burning and/or bleed-

ing occur, and determine and describe the kind, location, frequency, and duration of pain, and so on.)
6. If the patient does experience any difficulty with voiding, describe what he does to prevent and/or alleviate the difficulty.
7. Determine and note if the patient has a Foley catheter, colostomy, iliostomy, and so on.
C. Breathing
1. Observe and describe the patient's breathing. Include
   a. Whether the patient is mouth or nose breathing
   b. Whether the patient is chest or abdominal breathing
   c. Whether the breathing is audible or inaudible.
2. Describe any difficulty the patient experiences in breathing. In addition, note:
   a. When the patient experiences the difficulty
   b. That which influences the difficulty, i.e.,
      (1) Causes the difficulty or makes it worse
      (2) Relieves the difficulty.
3. Observe and note whether the patient is using oxygen, a respirator, Intermittent Positive Pressure Breathing (IPPB) machine, and so on.
D. Eating and drinking patterns
1. List each meal the patient eats, the time he eats the meal, and a typical menu.
   Example: Breakfast (0700) orange juice, egg, toast, and coffee.
2. Fluid intake:
   a. List the kinds of fluids the patient likes to drink.
   b. State the total amount of fluid the patient drinks daily.
3. State special dislikes, religious, and/or medical restrictions (special diet) the patient has related to food and/or fluid.
4. Describe any problems the patient has related to eating and drinking. Consider:
   a. Teeth, artificial dentures, ability to chew
   b. Swallowing, sight, ability to cut food, open containers, or to feed himself
   c. Nausea, vomiting, anorexia.
   Include:
      (1) How the problem affects the patient's ability to eat or drink
      (2) What he does about the problem
      (3) What assistance he needs.
5. Observe and note whether the patient has a nasogastric tube, gastrostomy tube, intravenous infusion for nutritional purposes, and so on.

E. Skin integrity
   1. Using the senses of touch and sight, describe the patient's skin in terms of:
      a. Color: pale, tan, ruddy, black, brown, yellow, blue, gray, pink
      b. Turgor: tight, firm, loose, wrinkled
      c. Texture: smooth, rough, scaly
      d. State: oily, dry, moist
   2. Observe and note the condition of the skin at the site of an incision, intravenous infusion, and so on.
   3. Examine the skin and describe any problems observed.
      a. Look at the bony prominences for redness or darkness (bony prominences include: the sacrum, coccyx, iliac spines, greater trochanters, heels, elbows, scapulae, the back of the head, and so on).
      b. Observe and describe any of the following: skin eruptions, decubiti, bruises, swelling, wounds, and scratches.
   4. Note what the patient says:
      a. He does to care for his skin
      b. About any skin problems he has
      c. He does to prevent or alleviate the skin problem, if he has one.
   5. Observe and describe the condition of the lips, tongue, and mucous membranes of the mouth.
   6. General hygiene
      a. Describe: (1) the frequency, (2) time of day, and (3) kind of bathing (tub bath, shower, partial bath, bed bath, and so on) the patient is accustomed to.
      b. Describe: (1) how often and (2) the time of day the patient usually shaves.
      c. State whether or not the patient is accustomed to wearing makeup.
      d. Describe how the patient is accustomed to caring for his teeth. Note:
         (1) Frequency and time(s) of day for cleaning teeth
         (2) Whether the patient wears dentures
         (3) If the patient has dentures, note whether he removes them or leaves them in place when sleeping.
      e. Note whether or not the patient needs assistance in any of the following areas. If he does, specify what the assistance consists of.
         (1) Bathing
         (2) Grooming (shaving, combing hair, and so on)
         (3) Mouth or denture care.

Example: Can partially bathe self; needs to have back, legs, and feet washed for him.

F. Activity
   1. Observe and describe the following:
      a. Ability to walk
      b. Range of joint motion.
      (*Note:* If, for a valid reason, these are not observed, state that you did not observe the patient to determine his ability to walk and/or his range of motion and describe what the patient says about his ability to walk and/or to move his joints through the complete range of motion.)
   2. Identify any limitation with either walking or range of motion. Include:
      a. The specific body part limited
      b. How it is limited
      c. How the limitation affects the patient's activities of daily living
      d. What assistance is needed due to the limitation.
   3. Note whether the patient uses any prosthesis or mechanical aid.

G. Recreation
   1. Describe what the patient usually does for recreation; for relaxation; how he spends his leisure time. Consider hobbies, special interests, and so on.

H. Interpersonal and communicative patterns
   1. Describe that which other people can do to help the patient feel more comfortable in a new situation or when he is with people he doesn't know.
   2. Describe the patient's nonverbal behavior during the interview. Include:
      a. Position (posture)
      b. Activity during the interview
      c. Anything significant about the patient's appearance (facial expression, grooming, clothing, and so on).
   3. Describe the patient's verbal behavior during the interview. Include:
      a. Answers or evades questions
      b. Volunteers or does not volunteer information
      c. Asks or does not ask questions
      d. Changes the subject or focus of the interview or conversation and/or jumps from topic to topic, or remains focused on the subject or topic of the interview
      e. Speaks clearly or indistinctly.

I. Temperament
  1. Describe those situations, things other people do, and so on, which tend to make the patient angry. Also include:
     a. A description of what the patient feels and/or what he does when he is angry
     b. How others know when he is angry.
J. Dependency and independency patterns
  (*Note:* This category is concerned with how the patient meets *both* his dependency *and* independency needs, *not* whether he is a dependent or independent person. This is based on the fact that people have both dependency and independency needs and ways of meeting both needs. It is essential to keep this in mind when eliciting information for this category.)
  1. Describe those ways in which the patient depends on others.
  2. Describe those ways in which others depend on the patient.
  3. Describe those experiences in which the patient has worked with others for mutual goals.
  4. Describe by example how the patient lets others know what he wants.
  5. Record how others can make the patient feel more comfortable about asking for and accepting help.
K. Senses
  1. Describe any problem the patient has related to sight. Include:
     a. How the problem affects him in terms of activities of daily living
     b. What others can do to assist him in this area.
  2. Note whether the patient wears glasses, contact lenses, or has an artificial eye.
  3. Describe any problem the patient has related to hearing. Include:
     a. How the problem affects him in terms of activities of daily living
     b. What others can do to assist him in this area.
  4. Note whether the patient uses a hearing aid.
  5. Note whether the patient is right or left handed.
L. Menstrual patterns
  1. State the usual frequency and duration of menstrual periods (or note that the patient has not reached menarche or has experienced menopause).
     a. Record the date of the patient's last menstrual period.
  2. Describe any difficulty the patient experiences in relation to menstruation (dysmenorrhea, amenorrhea, menorrhagia, metrorrhagia).
  3. If the patient does experience any difficulty, describe what she does to prevent and/or alleviate the difficulty.

27

VI. Statement of that which helps the patient feel cared for (i.e., secure, comfortable, protected, safe):
(*Note:* This category, as with others in the Nursing History, is concerned with what *usually* makes the patient feel cared for or secure, safe, comfortable, and protected. The usually is emphasized to mean before hospitalization, not what makes the patient feel cared for in the hospital.)
  A. Describe those items which are important to the patient (which usually tend to help him feel comfortable, secure, and so on).
  B. Describe those things others do, or have done in the past, which make the patient feel cared for.

RECORDING THE NURSING HISTORY

Any purpose for which the material may ultimately be used will be affected by the quality of the information recorded in the Nursing History. Therefore, the quality of the collected data must be of great concern if the information is to prove valuable. For this reason, and because this text is used for teaching nursing students, directions for writing the Nursing History are included. Allowing for some variations in details among institutions, practicing nurses and students are expected to record their Nursing Histories according to these directions and will be evaluated on this basis.

DIRECTIONS

1. Stamp the upper left space of the paper with the patient's addressograph.
2. Write the title "Nursing History" in the upper right space of the paper. This label should appear on each page of the history.
3. Write the date and time the history is taken. *Example:* 3-16-72 (1345)
4. Sign the Nursing History at the end. The signature is to include first initial, last name, and appropriate title. *Example:* B. Brown, R.N., or C. White, N.S.
5. Write across the entire page.
6. Write on both sides of the paper.
7. Begin a new line for each category (I through VI) and each subcategory (A through L within category V).
8. List each category and then record the pertinent data. *Example:* D. Eating and drinking patterns: breakfast (0730) juice, cereal, toast, 2 cups coffee. . . .
9. Record all the data considered to be "Baseline Data." (That list of data included earlier in this chapter.)
10. Write with a black ball-point pen.
11. Write the Nursing History at the "bedside."
The Nursing History must be written as the data is elicited. To take notes

or try to remember facts later makes the process infeasible in terms of nursing time and causes distortion, inaccuracy, and omission of valuable data. The history is put into the chart as it is written at the bedside, thus saving time and providing immediately available data. It is not to be rewritten before becoming part of the chart.

12. Follow the format of the Nursing History Guide to elicit and record the data. (See Appendix 1.)

13. Write in a telegraphic style.

This means that complete sentences are not always written. For example, the subject of the sentence may often be omitted without causing confusion, and articles (a, an, the) are not necessary. Simple phrases are sufficient. The intent is to be concise and specific, omitting unnecessary words. *Example:* 1) Bedtime—2030; awakens—0630. 2) Dislikes coffee. 3) B.M. q.d. within hour p̄ breakfast.

14. Use only acceptable medical abbreviations.

In other words, use only those abbreviations which are known to all persons concerned with the patient's chart. A list of acceptable abbreviations is included in Appendix 3. This list is not meant to include every abbreviation possible, only those used most frequently by nurses.

15. Spell correctly.

16. Use penmanship that can be read.

17. Use correct grammar.

While it is not necessary to write in complete sentences, the parts of speech used are to be grammatically correct. Use the correct tense of the verb, be consistent, and ascertain that the noun to which a pronoun refers is clearly understood.

18. Use short statements, choosing the simplest words possible which accurately convey the meaning. Cowan and McPherson make the following suggestions:[10]

a. A common, ordinary word is usually the best to use if there is a choice. "The word that everybody knows is the word that everybody is likely to understand."[11]

b. Use long and/or technical words only when necessary for precision. For example, use walk rather than ambulate, and talk rather than verbalize. Take care to find the right word for what is meant instead of some other word fairly close to it.

c. Use a word only when absolutely certain of its meaning.

d. Use new words when they really do make the meaning clearer, not for their sound.

19. Emphasize the relevant and minimize the irrelevant.

It may be difficult to recognize the relevant, especially for a beginning practitioner. However, as the nurse gains experience, she will become better able to differentiate between the relevant and the irrelevent. Examples of irrelevant data are: 1) the fact that the patient recently purchased a boat with no additional information as to the importance of this acquisition to the patient, or 2) the fact that the patient was wearing white pajamas and a blue and white robe with green slippers. In this last example, it would have been more relevant to note if the slippers fit so the patient would have no difficulty in walking. The intent is to record data that may be used in planning nursing care and the fact that a patient is wearing a blue robe is unlikely to aid in this.

20. Record the Nursing History as objectively as possible.

Before one can be objective, he must be able to distinguish between factual data and subjective data. Factual data is that which can be tested or checked using an accepted standard. Subjective data cannot be verified because it is based on opinions. For example, "The patient weighs 150 pounds" is a factual statement. It may not be precise, but it can be tested to determine its accuracy.[12] "The patient is thin" is a subjective statement. What does the recorder consider as "thin"? Thin in comparison with what standard? Subjective material is of little use to anyone other than the recorder. Since the data in the Nursing History is intended for use by many health professionals, it must be written in an objective, factual manner. Record only specific information, omitting such words as: small, good, some, usually, often, many. Do not make assumptions, interpretations, inferences as to causation, generalizations, or value judgments.

21. Record examples to support statements in the categories of Interpersonal and Communicative Patterns, Temperment, and Dependency and Independency Patterns. For example, in describing the temperment of a child, a nurse wrote, "Angry, impulsive toward adults." No data were recorded in the patient's chart to indicate the basis for such a statement. Another nurse recorded that a patient was "withdrawn." Again, no examples of this behavior were recorded. It is possible that the patient was simply disinterested or had a headache at the time. To avoid error, these statments should be clearly designated as hypotheses and tested to determine if they are a proper evaluation of the patient's behavior.

SUMMARY

The importance of obtaining objective, specific, and factual data cannot be overemphasized. Beveridge states that, "It is important not to confuse facts with their interpretations, that is to say, to distinguish between data and generalizations."[13] He goes on to say that scientists often make interpretations without realizing that they are departing from a statement of the facts. Willard states that, "Nurses who claim a scientific basis for their actions give the greatest priority to facts; they continually guard against making or accepting incomplete, ambiguous and erroneous statements. . . ."[14] The fact that this system requries high levels of selfdiscipline and frustration tolerance perhaps explains the opposition of many to its use. Nevertheless, it is an effective method of obtaining the high quality data necessary for planning care, teaching students, and defining research problems.

A NURSING HISTORY

The following example of a Nursing History demonstrates the format of the written history, the kind of data considered to be baseline data, and how this information is recorded. While this is an actual example of a history taken on a patient, all identifying information such as names, city of residence, and so on, have either been omitted or changed. This is also true of all other examples included in this text.

Addressograph   Nursing History

Stamp

1-21-72 (1430)

   I. Vital Statistics: First General Hospital admission for Mary Hunter, a 54 year old married woman from Little City, Fl.
  II. Patient's Understanding of Illness: Came to hospital due to "high blood pressure" and "fear that with the next breath I take I'm going to die." Feels "nervous" (meaning "about to go to pieces all the time") and "depressed" (cries, doesn't know what to do with her time, has gained 100 lbs. in 2 years). Began feeling depressed and nervous 2 years ago at which time her boss died of a "heart attack" and the business was bankrupt; patient lost job and stock held in the business. In next 2 months, father and 2 friends died of "heart attacks" and "Now I'm scared all the time that I'll have a heart attack and die." Was told that bed rest will keep blood pressure down so has remained in bed for the last month except to cook and eat. Feels weak (unsteady on feet).
 III. Patient's Expectations: Expects medication to lower blood pressure and "reassurance that nothing's wrong c̄ my heart." Expects to begin working (has to help c̄ bills) and to lose wt. Expects nurses to check blood pressure, tell her "it's all right" and to talk c̄ her.
 IV. Brief Social and Cultural History: Unemployed at present. Corporate secretary and office manager until 2 years ago. Had responsibility of seeing that others did their job. "That job meant a lot to me and now I have no job. Maybe that's my trouble." (Says she had not thought about loss of job attributing to illness before this.) Education—completed high school and law courses (business school). Had to go-to school to keep job. Family consists of husband and daughter. Lives c̄ husband. Says she always put daughter first until

31

daughter married last spring; says now husband is most significant person. Worried about finding job and paying bills.

V. Significant Data in Terms of:

A. Sleeping patterns: Goes to bed 1900 (nothing else to do); falls asleep 2200. Wakes up 0800–0900. Gets up at lunch time. When not sleeping thinks about being scared, what's going to happen to her, and how to get some help. Used to watch TV before going to bed but now TV makes her nervous. Wakes up in middle of night 4 or 5 times per week "starved to death." Eats apple, juice, or anything can find. After eating can return to sleep s̄ difficulty. Uses 1 pillow.

B. Eliminating patterns: B.M. q.d. p̄ breakfast. Last B.M. 1-20-72. Attributes maintenance of pattern to orange juice and hot coffee which she drinks q.d. for breakfast. Experiences no difficulty with bowels or voiding.

C. Breathing: At present, patient is nose breathing, using chest muscles and breathing is inaudible. Says when nervous (see category II) "my breath gets short," becomes frightened and "hyperventilates" (meaning breathes too fast). Breathing in paper sack helps. Says, "I get scared to death when this happens." Presently has dry cough; taking cough medicine per doctor's order. Smokes 2 packs/day; "I have to have a cigarette in my hand all the time."

D. Eating and drinking patterns: Breakfast (0800) coffee (3–4 cups between 0800 to noon) and orange juice; lunch (1200) 2 sandwiches, water or coffee; dinner (1700) steak, turnip greens, beans, cornbread. Fluid intake is approximately 2400 cc./day consisting of coffee, water, diet cola. Dislikes pork; no medical or religious restrictions. Tries not to eat potatoes or desserts. Eats at least 6 slices of bread/day. Has no problems eating or drinking. Eats more when upset, especially ice cream and candy, but may be anything can find.

E. Skin integrity: Skin is pale, loose, smooth, and dry. No redness or other skin problems observed. Cares for skin c̄ soap and water. Uses lotion for dryness of skin. Lips are dry and cracked; tongue furrowed; mucous membranes of mouth are dry. Ulcer ("very sore") approximately ⅛ inch in diameter in lower right mouth. Showers q.d. when gets up. Prefers tub bath but afraid to get in and out of tub by self. Used to wear makeup; none now. Brushes teeth (own) b.i.d., ā breakfast and h.s. Needs someone close by when showers as feels weak (unsteady), afraid of falling. Would like tub bath if could have help getting in and out of tub. Needs no other assistance.

F. Activity: Feels "weak and unsteady" on feet. "Head feels woozy all the time." Refused to walk alone. Observed to walk c̄ steady gait holding my arm but s̄ leaning on me. Observed to have full R.O.M. in all joints. No prostheses.

G. Recreation: "Loves" any kind of needlework, especially embroidery, but hasn't done anything but worry about self for 2 years.

H. Interpersonal and communicative patterns: No difficulty meeting people. Feels "ashamed and nervous" around any people since gaining wt. Afraid everyone will laugh at her. Doesn't go anywhere now as afraid will have "heart attack." Has no friends anymore. "Being c̄ people for any period of time makes me nervous." Is more comfortable if others come to her and not expect her to be "jolly like I was 2 years ago." Nonverbal behavior: sitting slumped on edge of bed one hand holding head (said head doesn't hurt—"I just feel depressed"). Smoking continuously. Looks depressed (face drawn, mouth turned downward, furrowed brow, cried whenever mentioning loss of appearance and job). Wearing wrinkled dress, no makeup, hair uncombed. Voice is soft, speaks slowly and in a monotone. Verbal behavior: answers and asks questions, volunteers information, speaks clearly, and keeps to the subject of the interview.

I. Temperament: Gets mad when husband leaves clothes laying around or tells her how to cook. When mad, "I bless him out." This makes patient nervous (shaky). Says "I used to get mad an awful lot but I found that it didn't help any." About loss of job and stocks, patient says she just felt depressed, like she had worked all those years "for nothing." Says it didn't make her mad, just depressed.

J. Dependency and independency patterns: Used to cook and sew for others; now does nothing. Says she's always done the helping; "No one's ever helped me c̄ anything." Doesn't want others to do anything for her; just relies on self. Says it feels "uncomfortable" to have others help her. "I don't know how to ask for help or how to accept it." Has to find a job to pay her share of the bills. "In our house nothing is ours. It's yours or mine." Patient and husband have agreement that she will pay certain bills and he will pay others. Says she's kept her end of the bargain by using her savings. Has money left for only one more month's bills, then doesn't know what will happen. Observation: When I offered to bring patient coffee, she replied, "Oh, would you?"

K. Senses: Wears glasses for reading and sewing. No problems hearing. Right handed.

L. Menstrual patterns: Postmenopause.

VI. That Which Helps Patient Feel Cared For: Has to have cigarettes.

Wants to find a job but doesn't know how to start all over. Was "proud" of her job. Says she used to be "perfect" in everything she did. "I did my job perfectly; my appearance was perfect." As long as worked, managed to keep wt. down; says, "Now look at me." Feels cared for when daughter calls q.d. Others thinking she did a good job used to make her feel "good."

D. Loring, R.N.

REFERENCES

1. *Webster's New Collegiate Dictionary.* G. and C. Merriam Company, Publishers, Springfield, 1960, p. 210.
2. Ibid., p. 72.
3. Weed, Lawrence L.: *Medical Records, Medical Education and Patient Care.* The Press of Case Western Reserve University, Cleveland, Year Book Medical Publishers, Inc., Chicago, 1969, p. 15.
4. Ibid., p. 72.
5. Bjorn, John C., and Cross, Harold D.: *The Problem-Oriented Private Practice of Medicine.* Modern Hospital Press, Chicago, 1970, p. 32.
6. Hurst, J. Willis, and Walker, H. Kenneth (eds.): *The Problem-Oriented System.* MEDCOM, Inc., New York, 1972.
7. Weed, Lawrence L.: "Questions often asked about the problem-oriented record—Does it guarantee quality?" in Hurst, J. W., and Walker, H. K. (eds.): *The Problem-Oriented System.* MEDCOM, Inc., New York, 1972, p. 54.
8. Bjorn and Cross, *op. cit.*, p. 596.
9. Randall, R. Beauvais: "Errors frequently made in using the problem-oriented system," in Hurst, J. W., and Walker, H. K. (eds.): *The Problem-Oriented System.* MEDCOM, Inc., New York, 1972, p. 68.
10. Cowan, Gregory, and McPherson, Elisabeth: *Plain English Please.* Random House, New York, 1966, pp. 112–114.
11. Ibid., p. 112.
12. Ibid., pp. 116, 117.
13. Beveridge, W. I. B.: *The Art of Scientific Investigation,* third edition. W. W. Norton and Company, Inc., New York, 1957, p. 87.
14. Willard, Marian C.: "A matter of facts." *Nursing Outlook* 11:832, 1963.

4

THE COLLECTION OF DATA

The development of an adequate technique for making sound observations and for taking a reliable and useable Nursing History is the primary skill a nurse can acquire to assure success in the present practice of clinical nursing. A practitioner can no longer depend upon the adaptation of social conversation to professional situations, but must master specific principles and techniques useful in the collection of data. Unless she feels comfortable and is competent in gathering data, she will practice with incomplete information for which no other skill can compensate.[1] Data is collected from a patient to help know him as a person as well as to ascertain information necessary to plan and deliver effective, safe, and comforting nursing care. This requires data about the patient's life-style, usual patterns, and customary practices for coping with his activities of daily living. In addition, information is needed to identify those problems which the patient can no longer manage or solve for himself and to determine whether these are a result of his lack of necessary strength, will, or knowledge. Finally, data are needed in order to write a plan of care and to evaluate and update the plan. Therefore, this chapter presents general guidelines applicable to the collection of data from and about patients. Emphasis is placed on the interview as a means of collecting this information, and on the initial interview for obtaining the Nursing History in particular. However, the reader will hopefully find these guidelines useful throughout the entire process of working with and caring for patients.

OBSERVATION

Observation is defined here as a method of gathering data by noticing and recording facts or occurrences. It is not limited exclusively to sight, but involves the other senses as well. It is an active mental process consisting of two elements: the sensory perception element, and the mental element.[2] This involves perceiving something, recording the perception, and attaching significance to it.

Observation is selective and may be influenced by both conscious and unconscious factors. Smith states:

1. We observe what we want to observe.
2. We observe what we expect to observe.
3. We observe what we have learned to observe.
4. What we are observing can change without our ever knowing it.[3]

There are two types of observations: 1) spontaneous (passive) observations which are unexpected, and 2) induced (active) observations which are deliberately sought, usually in relation to a hypothesis.

Effective, spontaneous observation involves. . .noticing some object or event. The thing noticed will only become significant if the mind of the observer either consciously or unconsciously relates it to some relevant knowledge or past experience, or if in pondering on it subsequently he arrives at some hypothesis. . . .[4]

The intellectual skill of observation is one that can be developed with conscious direction. The observer must become aware of how much he doesn't notice and then identify the things he repeatedly misses. Individual patterns of selective observation are determined by preferences, alertness, range and depth of knowledge, and the goals sought.[5] According to Mumford and Skipper:

Scientists train themselves to see more, and more accurately, in their special fields. Prepared through intensive interest and study, some have come upon discoveries because they could take note of and make new sense of what many other men had been exposed to and missed. Science starts with observation and has to return to observation for validation.[6]

INTERVIEW

The interview has been defined in a variety of ways. The definition that best describes the kind of interviewing used in this system of nursing practice is:

A specialized pattern of verbal interaction—initiated for a specific purpose, and focused on some specific content area, with subsequent elimination of extraneous material. Moreover, the interview is a pattern of interaction in which the role relationship of the interviewer and respondent is highly specialized, its specific characteristics depending somewhat on the purpose and character of the interview.[7]

The interview may be utilized:

1. To secure information from people,

2. To give information to people, and/or
3. To influence the behavior of people.[8]

Types of Interviews

For use with this clinical tool, two types of interviews are advocated: the information-getting interview, and the helping interview. While the techniques used in both are similar, the conduct and focus differ. Most interviews are a combination of both types; however, early nurse-patient interactions are more often used to obtain data and later ones to give the patient information necessary for managing his nursing problems.

THE INFORMATION-GETTING INTERVIEW

This is the type of interview used in obtaining the Nursing History. It is structured and controlled in that the topics discussed are predetermined by the defined data base. The structured interview has proven a more effective and efficient method of gathering data than the unstructured type, yielding about twice the amount of information in approximately half the time it takes to conduct an unstructured interview.[9]

It is the nurse's responsibility to obtain all necessary information and, in the interest of efficiency, limit extraneous conversation. "It is in this sense that the interaction in an information-getting interview is controlled...."[10] However, the information-getting interview is by no means restricted to superficial or easily verbalized data. As Kahn and Cannell state:

[It] attempts to get at partially formed attitudes and at private, seldom-verbalized feelings. The interviewer may even contribute, through his techniques and the relationship he establishes, to the respondent's ability to formulate and pull together his attitudes regarding the topic under discussion.[11]

This is not to imply that the information-getting interview is a psychiatric interview. It is not intended to delve deeply into the personality structure of the patient or uncover material which has been kept at an unconscious level. Also, this type of interview is not designed to change the patient. "Indeed, it is the absence of the intent to change which perhaps most sharply differentiates the information-getting interview from a variety of other kinds of interview situations."[12]

THE HELPING INTERVIEW

This type of interview is used to give information to the patient or to influence or change his behavior when necessary for the management of his nursing problems. It is an unstructured type of interview, as opposed to the structured type used in the information-getting situation. There are no uniform, predetermined topics to be discussed; the patient is encouraged to choose his own subjects and speak freely.

The Interview Process

If conducted properly, the interview can be a powerful tool to obtain accurate and otherwise unavailable material. However, improper interviewing can seriously restrict the flow of communication or yield distorted information. According to Bingham and Moore:

The ability to interview rests not on any single trait, but on a vast complex of them. Habits, skills, techniques, and attitudes are all involved. Competence in interviewing is acquired only after careful and diligent study, prolonged practice (preferably under supervision), and a good bit of trial and error; for interviewing is not an exact science; it is an art.[13]

The interview process consists of four major phases:

1. Preparation
2. Initiation
3. Direction
4. Termination.

These phases and techniques common to each for the collection of data are discussed below. These guidelines are organized according to the stage of the interview in which they are most commonly utilized. However, when appropriate, they can be employed in other phases. While these techniques do not guarantee successful interviews, they generally facilitate collection of accurate, complete data and establishment of an effective nurse-patient relationship.

PREPARATION

Adequate preparation can greatly enhance the manner in which the interview is conducted. When preparing for the interview, the nurse should bear in mind the three basic ingredients essential to any successful interview: 1) establishment of rapport with the patient, 2) formation of specific interview objectives, and 3) formulation of questions which fulfill the objectives.[14]

Establishing *rapport* involves building a relationship characterized by harmony and confidence. This is facilitated by a friendly, courteous, interested approach and acceptance of the patient's attitudes and ideas without expression of moral or ethical judgments.[15]

38

The nurse must form specific objectives to be achieved by the interview. Since these goals determine the communication which occurs, *the interview conducted by the nurse is said to be goal-directed.* Thus, it is necessary for the nurse to know clearly what she wishes to accomplish within a particular interview. She must be able to obtain the desired information and exclude irrelevant material. In a successful interview, communication takes place frankly and freely, and since the interview is goal-directed, the content is focused and controlled so that the initial purpose of the interview is achieved. *The interview must always remain focused on particular "content objectives."* [16]

The content objectives define the precise kinds of information that will be needed to meet the purpose for which the interview is held. They form the links between the general purpose of the interview and the specific questions which the nurse asks. If the collection of a defined data base is part of the assessment process, the content objectives are already identified. However, it is no small matter for the nurse to thoroughly familiarize herself with this defined data base and the information required to complete it.

The nurse must also formulate content objectives for later interactions with the patient (those taking place after the defined data base has been collected). Therefore, in preparing for the interaction, she must decide the precise kinds of information to be obtained within a particular time period. This is not to imply that only predetermined information is obtained from the interview. While most patients volunteer much valuable data, the nurse cannot depend upon them to volunteer all the necessary information. Thus, it is the nurse's responsibility to determine that all major topics are included and that the defined data base is collected.

The purpose of the interview and the specific content objectives guide the choice of the questions to be asked. While the content objectives specify the kinds of information to be obtained during the interview, they do not tell how to formulate the questions needed to elicit the desired information. They merely remind the nurse of what is wanted, but do not tell her how to get it. It cannot be stressed too often that the content objectives are not the questions to be asked during the interview.

The primary purpose of interview questions is to communicate the specific content objectives in such a manner that they can be understood by the patient. They must convey the kind of information required, and lead to responses which fulfill the objectives.

Since the interviewer is asking questions, the type of interaction he achieves will depend to a considerable extent on the quality of the questions he asks. Skillfully worded questions can do a great deal to assist and guide the interviewer in developing respondent motivation to communicate. [17]

While preparing to interview the patient, the nurse should consider the information to be collected and determine alternate questions or methods for obtaining it. However, she should not use a list of these questions while conducting the interview as this encourages dependency upon a limited number of methods and may cause her to panic if the information is not readily obtained. Rather, the nurse should familiarize herself with various methods and be able, during the interview, to choose an alternative means of obtaining the data.

There are primarily three decisions which the interviewer must make in preparing adequate questions for fulfilling objectives and motivating communication:

1. *The choice of words.* The nurse must ask her questions so that the patient can understand them.
2. *Whether to ask an "open" or "closed" question.* The nurse decides whether to ask a question so that the patient is restricted to choosing his answer from a prearranged list of choices or by "yes" or "no," or so that he must answer in his own words.
3. *The choice between a direct or an indirect approach to a particular objective.*[18]

These are discussed later in this chapter under "Direction of the Interview."

Taking time to adequately prepare for an interview will make it a more enjoyable and profitable experience for both patient and nurse. The nurse will perform better and with more confidence when she feels prepared, and this transmits a feeling of security to the patient.

INITIATION

When taking a Nursing History, as in most nurse-patient situations, the nurse initiates the interaction with the patient. *There are specific techniques which the nurse can use to initiate the interaction.* The manner in which the nurse approaches the patient and the interview situation determines the way in which the patient responds to her and her attempts to obtain information. Brammer and Shostrom say that, "Ordinary human courtesy goes far toward establishing rapport with the patient."[19]

Before meeting the patient, the nurse should learn his name and proper title. She can then greet him by name, making him feel more comfortable. This also tells him that the nurse has made an attempt to find out about him and is acknowledging his individuality. Other suggestions for helping the patient become more comfortable with the interview situation include a smile, a handshake, and the offer of coffee, tea, water, or juice if it is available and not contraindicated. A few general but friendly remarks about such topics as where the patient is from, whether this is his first time in this particuar hospital, or comments or questions about pictures or flowers in his room are also useful when initiating a relationship with the patient. These topics are familiar, easy to talk about, and nonthreatening to most people. Starting with topics such as these helps the patient feel more comfortable with the nurse and the interview situation, and thus helps him talk about other matters.

The manner in which the nurse presents herself to the patient influences his perception of her and her professional role. The nurse should always introduce herself, making certain that she includes: her name, position, purpose for being there, and the approximate length of time she plans to be with the patient. When the nurse or student presents herself as a responsible person involved with the team that will be caring for him, the patient will generally readily accept her as a member of the professional staff and be more than willing to cooperate and seek her help with meeting his needs and solving his problems. The introduction may be accompanied by a handshake. This is a familiar gesture to most people and provides a way of initiating physical contact. However, physical contact makes some patients uncomfortable and in these cases should be avoided whenever possible. Offering to shake hands gives the nurse a clue as to how the patient feels about physical contact with another person, since he can always choose to ignore her offer. Information can also be obtained from the manner in which he shakes hands. However, the nurse should not form hasty conclusions about the patient's feelings or misinterpret her own discomfort as his. Physical contact as an aid to communication is also discussed later in this chapter under "Direction of the Interview."

There is specific information which the patient should be given about the interview. The patient must be able to perceive some benefit for himself resulting from his participation in the interview. The patient may be motivated to fulfill his responsibility in the interaction if he clearly understands the following:

1. The purpose of the interview
2. The ways in which the information he contributes is to be used
3. What will be expected of him during the interview.[20,21]

The nurse should explain to the patient that the purpose of the interview is to obtain particular information about him for use in providing the best possible nursing care. His preferences and usual patterns will be considered when planning his care and maintained whenever feasible. In order to achieve this, the nurse will ask him specific questions and record his responses. The patient is requested to reply to the best of his ability; if he has any questions or does not understand what is wanted he should not hesitate to ask the nurse.

The setting the nurse creates for the interview serves to facilitate or inhibit communication. The nurse can use skill and imagination in making the interview setting as comfortable as possible for the patient. This helps establish rapport, which in turn facilitates communication. Several of the numerous techniques which the nurse may employ are discussed below.

The nurse must allow sufficient time, free from interruptions, to complete the interview. If either the nurse or patient feels hurried, neither participant will give the situation his or her best. The nurse should arrange the time of the interview with the staff so that it does not conflict with medication or treatment schedules or their effects, and to eliminate unnecessary interruptions. Visiting hours should also be avoided as a time for conducting the interview.

The patient should be provided as much privacy as possible during the interview. This is aided by closing the door of a private room, or drawing the curtains around the bed in a nonprivate room. This lessens the possibility of being overheard or interrupted, eliminates distractions, and provides an atmosphere of confidentiality. The nurse should keep the volume of her voice not louder than that necessary for the patient to hear her.

The nurse should do everything possible to ensure the patient's and her own comfort during the interview. Attending to such measures as positioning the patient, pouring a glass of water, helping him to the bathroom, or obtaining an extra blanket communicates to the patient that the nurse is genuinely concerned about his well-being. A comfortable patient who feels cared for by the nurse will contribute more readily to the interview than an uncomfortable one.

The nurse should sit near the patient where he can easily see and communicate with her. Her sitting indicates that he is important; she is taking time to talk with and listen to him and will not be leaving at any moment. She should also face the patient and look at him when he or she is speaking. This re-enforces his identity as an individual person, not merely a form to be completed.

DIRECTION

It is the nurse's responsibility to guide the course of the interview by means of her responses and questions. Some patients require much direction from the nurse and others very little; however, all require some degree of guidance if the defined data base is to be gathered or if the content objectives for later interviews are to be achieved. The material in this section specifies guidelines and techniques for effective interviewing.

General Guidelines

Begin with those topics which are easiest for the patient to discuss. The sequence of interview questions should progress from least to most personal. Vanderzanden and Vanderzanden state:

If the nurse begins with questions that the patient can answer and that he is willing to answer, confidence can be gained, resentment minimized, and cooperation furthered through establishing the habit and attitude of answering.[22]

According to Kahn and Cannell, opening questions must be such that:

1. The patient can answer them without difficulty
2. The patient learns from them what his role is
3. They help the patient reassure himself that he can successfully play the role expected of him
4. They get the interview started successfully.[23]

Limit questions to a single idea or reference and ask only one question at a time. This helps prevent the patient from becoming confused and eliminates the problem of determining which part of the question he is answering at any given time.

Ask a short question rather than a long one. If a question is too long, the patient may become confused or stop listening altogether. Also, he may forget or simply ignore some of the qualifications to be considered when answering.

Use language that the patient can understand. Patients may respond to questions giving inaccurate information rather than admit that they do not understand a term used by the nurse. Also, the patient may not interpret the question in the same manner as the nurse. She must be alert to the fact that many terms have different meanings to different people. The nurse must scrutinize her wording to avoid ambiguity and/or language the patient does not understand. While the language of the interview must conform to the shared vocabulary of the nurse and the patient, this does not mean that she should use the same colloquialisms, expressions, and inflections as the patient. As Vanderzanden and Vanderzanden state:

Attempting to imitate these characteristics might seriously offend the patient. . . . The patient is bound to realize that any such efforts are unusual in the behavior of the nurse and may easily conclude that he is somehow being patronized.[24]

Allow sufficient time for the patient to answer. The nurse must use her judgment regarding how much time is sufficient. Based upon the patient's nonverbal clues, she must decide whether the patient is merely thinking about his answer or having difficulty with the question. It is possible that the patient did not hear or understand the question, or that it made him uncomfortable. The nurse should question the patient to determine his problem, and then decide how best to proceed.

Attend to the verbal and nonverbal signals from the patient. A successful interview depends upon the interviewer picking up on verbal leads and nonverbal signals from the patient.[25] These may include particular words

43

or themes which the patient uses repeatedly or certain statements which he makes more emphatically than others. By noting such signals the nurse can identify problems and/or clues that need to be followed up. This procedure often uncovers a single theme that explains many seemingly unrelated behaviors. For example, a patient may cry each time she mentions the death of her husband, and date changes in her physiologic and psychologic habit patterns or activities to his death. Thus, one of this patient's nursing problems would be grief concerning her husband's death. However, the nurse should not attempt an in-depth investigation at the time of the initial interview for two basic reasons. First, she has only begun to establish a relationship with the patient and it may be too early for the patient to lower her defenses and reveal the true extent of her grief. Second, the nurse needs particular data to begin caring adequately for the patient and which may enable her to help the patient express and deal with her grief.

Learn to become aware of one's own nonverbal communication and utilize it to facilitate the progress made during the interview. In any interpersonal situation, including the interview, much more may be communicated by nonverbal means (movements, gestures, and body posture) than by words. Benjamin states:

A gesture on the interviewer's part may communicate: "Yes, I'm with you, go on." or "I'm waiting, sensing that you have not finished." or . . . "I'm beginning to get bored." Our gestures mean much, so do our glances and the way we move about in our chair.[26]

According to Greenhill, nonverbal effectiveness includes:

1. Emphasizing physical proximity to the patient
2. Timing closer proximity to support the patient when he is exploring emotionally charged areas
3. Using minimal motor activity
4. Maintaining an accepting and nonpunitive attitude.[27]

The nurse must develop an awareness of her own nonverbal behavior in order to purposefully utilize it during the interview.

Maintain contact with the patient during the interview as a means of encouraging communication. There are many ways in which the nurse may achieve this, both verbally and nonverbally. Some examples are: nodding her head, changing facial expressions, altering her posture, and making occasional comments such as "I understand." or "Is that so?" when appropriate. These activities may be used to:

1. Let the patient know that the nurse comprehends what he is saying, is interested, and is listening.
2. Tell the patient that the nurse thinks that he is participating adequately in the interview and is "doing what is expected of him."

3. Indicate to the patient that the nurse would like him to continue speaking on the same topic.
4. Encourage the patient to continue speaking without specifying the scope or direction of the further response.[28]

Utilize physical contact as a means of facilitating communication. The use of touch, while largely ignored, is a significant communication channel between nurse and patient which can greatly strengthen their verbal interaction. Durr reports that:

Physical contact as a means of communication between nurse and patient was seen by patients as having several dimensions: giving direction, providing reinforcement of verbal encouragement, reducing fear, transmitting feelings of interest and concern, and demonstrating commitment to individuals in their recovery efforts.[29]

During the interview, the use of touch can be especially useful in helping the patient express difficult material. A touch on his hand or arm may give him the encouragement he needs to continue. On occasions when the patient begins to cry during the interview, it is most helpful for the nurse to stay close by, saying nothing, but perhaps placing her hand on the patient's hand, arm, or shoulder. In addition to comforting the patient, the nurse's touch tells him that it is acceptable to cry, that the nurse is willing to wait until he can continue, and may, by itself, encourage the patient to talk because of the feeling of concern he derives from her communication.

Ask questions in such a manner that they cannot be answered by "Yes" or "No." This avoids needless repetition, and keeps time, effort, and frustration to a minimum. For example, asking "Do you have any trouble chewing your food?" will obtain a yes or no answer. If the patient says "Yes," the nurse must then formulate additional questions to define the problem. Also, the initial approach "Tell me about your chewing difficulties" may only serve to offend the patient if he does not have problems in this area. In order to obtain all the desired information in answer to a single question, the nurse should say, "Please describe what, if any, difficulties you have chewing food." Other examples of this technique include asking "What formal education have you received?" rather than "Did you finish high school?" and "Tell me what your pain feels like" rather than "Is the pain sharp?"

Keep the interview focused on the topic under consideration until the required data have been obtained. The patient may tend to digress. When necessary, ask a question or make a suggestion which will lead the patient back to the appropriate topic. For example, the nurse may remark, "Before we discuss your weight problem, there is still some information I need about your sleeping difficulties. You were saying. . . ."

It is equally important to *move on to the next topic or question once the data has been elicited.* As soon as a question is satisfactorily answered, the nurse should begin to concentrate on the next question. This does not mean that she forgets what she has learned from the patient, merely that she does not hinder the progress of the interview by lingering unnecessarily on completed topics.

Inappropriately changing the topic of conversation is a problem which usually results from the nurse's inattentiveness, inability to identify the significance of the patient's conversation, preoccupation with other matters, and/or inability to control her own anxiety. For example, if the patient says "I'm afraid I won't live through the operation," it is inappropriate for the nurse to change the subject by responding "It's time to take your medicine." It is the nurse's responsibility to help the patient explore his fears, express them freely, and receive any information, suggestions, and assistance from her which will enable him to better handle these feelings. She must overcome her own anxiety concerning the subject of death in order to provide for the needs of the patient.

Obtain specific answers. Do not be content with vague answers. When the patient uses terms such as sometimes, often, little, and much, clarify what is meant by them and record only this specific information. A response which is open to more than one interpretation does not supply the data necessary to plan effective nursing care.

Utilize data previously elicited from the patient. Data already obtained from the patient can be used to suggest or facilitate further questions. For example, in the early part of the interview the patient frequently includes references to physiologic and/or psychologic patterns. He may say that his pain keeps him from sleeping, or that he cannot eat without becoming nauseated. When the interview progresses to the categories of sleep and eating, the nurse can begin by alluding to the patient's previous statements. This will show the patient that she has been listening and will serve to introduce the new category. In addition, correlation of the patient's prehospitalization patterns to his present situation may help obtain new data about the patient's attitudes, feelings, and thoughts regarding these changes.

Use some transitional comment when moving from one category to the next. Transitional comments are used to inform the patient that discussion of a certain topic has been completed and the nurse will proceed to the next subject. Thus, the focus of the interview can be redirected smoothly and effectively. The nurse may decide to change the topic of discussion because:

1. She has obtained all the information she needs pertaining to a particular topic.
2. She feels that the patient has nothing further to say.
3. She feels that the patient is uncomfortable, embarrassed, or threatened by the subject matter to the point that additional questioning would seriously affect further progress in the interview or

even the entire nurse-patient relationship. (In this instance the nurse may always return to the topic at a later time during the interview or during later interactions with the patient when he seems more capable of discussing it.)[30]

In the last instance, the nurse must ascertain that she is not prematurely changing the topic and that it is the patient's discomfort she is responding to and not her own.

The ability to make satisfactory transitions from one subject to another is an important facet of interviewing. In this manner, the nurse can choose the next topic she wishes to discuss with the patient and effect its introduction. If the subject is changed abruptly without proper transition, the patient may feel stranded. Examples of transitional statements include:

1. Summarizing what the patient has said previously and then making a statement such as, "That leads to the subject of. . . ."
2. "You have given me the information I need about your eating patterns and now I would like to discuss your sleeping patterns."
3. "When we were discussing your illness, you mentioned having difficulty sleeping. Well, I'd like to talk with you now about your sleeping patterns."

Specific Techniques

There are specific techniques the nurse can use to direct the interview. Many of these pertain to methods of questioning, and in order to use them effectively the nurse must first understand the various purposes for which questions can be used. According to Kahn and Cannell, questions have two primary purposes:

1. To provide the means by which the interviewer may obtain the information needed to fulfill the content objectives (in this case, to collect the defined data base)
2. To assist the interviewer to motivate the patient to communicate freely.[31]

However, there are several other, more specific purposes than these.

1. Questions may help the nurse focus the interview on the specific topic about which she needs information. Thus, the question guides the patient's attention to particular information.
2. The right question at the right time may help the patient to talk more freely about a specific topic. Questions communicate interest and an attempt to understand what the patient has to say. Thus encouraged, the patient is better able to express his thoughts, feelings, and ideas.

47

3. The question may be used to assist the patient to clarify or further explore a thought, feeling, or idea by providing the structure he needs in order to continue.
4. Questions may be used in order to obtain additional information needed to better understand what the patient is saying and/or to collect the defined data base. Questions are frequently used because we have part, but not all, of the necessary information pertaining to a content objective.
5. A question can be used to assist a patient who is having difficulty answering a previous question; it can end an awkward silence.

Based on an understanding of what can be accomplished through questions, the nurse can more effectively employ the various techniques discussed below.

Open and closed questions. The open question is a broad, less restricted question, giving greater freedom to the patient (and less control to the interviewer), in the sense that he is expected to reply in his own words. It simply establishes the topic for the patient and allows him to structure his answer as he sees fit. Open questions are used to solicit the patient's views, opinions, thoughts, and feelings. The closed question is a narrow, restricted question, offering the patient the least freedom (and the interviewer the greatest control), in that he is limited to a specific choice of answers. It requires the patient to select the answer that best approximates his own opinion from a group of responses given to him by the nurse.

Closed Questions	*Open Questions*
Do you prefer coffee or tea?	What do you like to drink?
Do you like to read?	How do you spend the time when you're not working?
Is the pain sharp?	Tell me what the pain is like.

Direct and indirect questions. Direct questions are straight and to the point. They may be open or closed questions. The indirect question asks a question without seeming to do so. It may serve to make an open question more open. While it may not have a question mark at the end of it, it is evident that a question is being asked and an answer sought.

Direct Questions	*Indirect Questions*
What keeps you awake at night?	It must be difficult to be unable to sleep at night. What kinds of things to you think about while you're awake?
How do you feel about having the operation?	I've been wondering about the feelings you might have now that your surgery has been scheduled.

Primary and secondary questions. The primary question is any question used to introduce a new topic or to ask for new content. Regardless of the care with which the nurse has worded a question, the patient's initial response may not be complete in terms of obtaining the desired information. At these times, the nurse must employ a secondary question. This is intended to elicit more fully the desired information by supplying additional focus and direction. The secondary question must enable the interviewer to:

1. Motivate additional communication on the required topic
2. Enhance or at least maintain the interpersonal relationship with the patient
3. Be able to accomplish both items listed above without introducing bias or modifying the meaning of the primary question.[32]

The following example illustrates the primary and secondary question.

Nurse: What happened to make you come to the hospital at this time? (primary question)
Patient: I started having more trouble with my arthritis.
Nurse: Tell me what kind of trouble you are having. (secondary question)

Clarification. Clarification seeks to elucidate replies which are vague, incomplete, or not meaningful.[33] The nurse must consider each response carefully and determine whether or not it answers her question, whether she needs further information to clarify the patient's answer, and whether she is indeed certain of what the patient meant by his answer or by any term he uses.

The nurse is responsible for directing and maintaining effective communication during the interview. Thus, she must determine that both she and the patient attach the same meanings to the words they use. Complete, specific information is necessary to provide the patient with the best possible nursing care. Also, upon realizing that he has been misunderstood, the patient may wonder why the nurse pretended to understand him and interpret this as a lack of interest or concern on her part. Therefore, much of the nurse's effort during the interview must be directed toward clarification of patient responses. Examples of words which almost always need clarification include: small, some, usually, often, many, seizures, spells, weak, nervous, and depressed. Once the patient has explained what he means by a certain term the nurse should not continue to seek clarification each time it is used. She may occasionally state, "You mean . . . ." thereby letting him know that she remembers. However, this should be done selectively, not repeatedly. While not its primary purpose, seeking clarification may have the secondary benefit of letting the patient know that the nurse is listening and trying to understand him and what he has to say. Some examples are:

"I didn't understand what you were just saying. Would you explain it again?"

"I'm sorry, I don't understand what you mean by trouble with your legs. Try telling me just what the trouble is."

Focusing statements or questions. Focusing is a technique used to control the interaction or conversation between the nurse and the patient by concentrating it on the content objectives for the interview or on a particular topic or question. According to Kahn and Cannell:

[Focusing] serves to increase the efficiency and effectiveness of the interaction by instructing the respondent as to what is relevant and irrelevant, thereby reducing or eliminating the communication of material which would not serve the purposes for which the interview was initiated.[34]

Focusing can be used when the patient talks about the correct subject but doesn't answer the specific question asked of him, or when he changes the topic of the conversation. As an example of the former situation, suppose that the nurse asked the patient to describe the kinds of things that make him angry and the patient talks about getting angry and losing control of oneself being wrong. The nurse may reply, "Mr. Brown, you've told me how you feel about people becoming angry. All people have some things they don't like or that they find irritating. What are these things for you?" In the latter situation, the nurse may refocus the interview by stating, for example, "Before we talk about that, tell me more about the times you have trouble breathing." The nurse may also use focusing to help the patient identify and express his thoughts and feelings about what he has been saying. Examples of this use include: "How did that make you feel?" and "What thoughts did you have when your boss said you couldn't work anymore until you saw a doctor?"

Reflection. There are two general categories of reflection techniques: 1) the reflection of content, and 2) the reflection of feelings.[35] The first category involves reflecting (or repeating) certain words or phrases spoken by the patient. This is sometimes referred to as "restating" or "echoing." The reflection of content may be achieved in the following ways: 1) Restating exactly what the patient has said, changing only the pronoun. (Patient: I've been trying to make a decision. Nurse: You've been trying to make a decision. 2) Restating part of what the patient has said, the part the nurse feels to be most significant. (Patient: I've been worried about my job. Nurse: Worried?) This lets the patient hear what he has said on the assumption that it may encourage him to think about it and continue talking. Also, this technique demonstrates that the nurse has listened to

50

what the patient has said and is willing to explore the subject further with him.

The second category of reflection pertains to feelings, attitudes, or impressions of behavior perceived regarding the patient. The reflection of feelings is sometimes referred to as "mirroring." When the nurse observes a particular behavior exhibited by the patient, she can verbalize her impression of what the behavior seems to communicate. For example, if the nurse observes that the patient has been pacing in his room all morning, she may say, "You seem to be more nervous today, Mr. Jones." or "I've noticed that you have been walking back and forth across your room all morning, Mr. Jones." When the nurse perceives a particular feeling communicated in the patient's statement, she can respond to that feeling rather than to what the patient has said. For example, if the patient says, "I have to keep coming back here for more treatments. I'm so tired of it; I'm thinking there's no use." the nurse may say, "You sound discouraged, Mr. Jones." The feeling perceived by the nurse may be expressed verbally as a means of telling the patient that the nurse has been listening, has some understanding of what the patient is saying, and is encouraging him to continue talking about the particular topic.

A common mistake made in using the reflective technique is the repetitive use of the introductory phrase, "You feel. . . ." This can arouse feelings of resentment, rendering the technique ineffective. Brammer and Shostrom suggest the following variety of introductory phrases:

Use of the word that expresses the feeling, such as "You were mad (sorry, confused, etc.) when that happened."
"You think . . ."
"You believe . . ."
"It seems to you . . ."
"As I get it, you feel that . . ."
"In other words . . ."
". . . is that it?"
"I gather that . . ."
Inflection or intonation of various words to express the reflection.[36]

According to Brammer and Shostrom, reflection may be used immediately after a statement has been made by the patient, as a summary, or as a terminating technique. Immediate reflection involves verbalizing the word or phrase immediately after it has been stated or implied by the patient. Summary reflection consists of briefly restating several statements or feelings which have been expressed by the patient. Terminal reflection is used to summarize the important aspects of the entire interview period.[37]

Reflection of feeling is one of the most important techniques for promoting a feeling of understanding. It is also one of the most difficult, requiring the ability to recognize and state the feelings and attitudes underlying the patient's words. It is important that the interviewer remember that the reflection of feelings involves responding only to the feeling tone of the patient, not to his own inner frame of reference. Brammer and Shostrom state that:

It takes considerable skill to develop the sensitivity necessary to identify these feelings immediately and to mirror them back as soon as the client has completed his statements.[38]

When the nurse reflects the patient's feeling or statement, the patient may either reject the nurse's statement or pick up on the reflected statement and continue talking. Usually, however, the reflected statement will be accepted by the patient because it merely consists of putting into words the feeling tone of what he has already expressed.[39]

Summarizing statements or questions. Summarizing is a technique which organizes and restates briefly the important points of what the patient has said. It can be used to increase clarity, specificity, or coherence of a response or of a series of responses.[40] In this way the nurse can omit irrelevant material and organize the pertinent aspects of the interview.[41]

Summarizing lets the patient hear succinctly from the nurse what she has understood him to have said. This allows the patient to verify that the interviewer has correctly understood what he was trying to communicate. If the patient finds that the summarization does not represent accurately or completely what he wanted to say, he is then in a position to reword his answer so as to make himself understood. Thus, misunderstandings and failures in communication can often be corrected. However, as Richardson and others point out, there is a risk to be considered when using this technique. As with other closed questions, it is often easier for the patient to agree with the nurse's summary than to disagree with it. This is especially true if the summary has been used to clarify ambiguous information.[42] The nurse should directly ask the patient if this (the summary) is what he meant. For example, she could preface the summary with a statement such as, "Let's see if I understood you correctly. I'll say what I think you said and you make whatever corrections are needed."

Summarizing is often helpful if used before proceeding to a new topic or question. The nurse may summarize what the patient has said, ask if this statement is accurate, make any necessary corrections, and then introduce the new topic. In this way, summarizing facilitates the transition from one topic to another. (Refer to the previous section on transitions in this chapter.) Summarizing may also be used to provide the reassurance and encouragement necessary to stimulate further communication, to coordinate seemingly unrelated pieces of information and thus aid in determining their significance, and to control the interview by limiting irrelevant conversation.

Silence. In the information-getting interview, silence may be used:

52

1. To indicate to the patient that the nurse expects him to speak
2. To give the patient an opportunity to organize his thoughts, recall the information requested, or think through a point
3. To direct the patient's thoughts to the task at hand—consideration of the question
4. To give the nurse an opportunity to observe the patient's nonverbal communication
5. To give the nurse time to record information, consider alternative ways of asking a question, or decide what she wants to ask next.

In addition to the above reasons, silence may be employed in a helping interview:

1. To allow the patient to take the initiative for the conversation
2. To give the patient time to consider alternative courses of action, explore his feelings, or make a decision
3. To enable the patient to discover that he can be accepted even though he doesn't feel like talking at the time.

The positive utilization of silence as a technique for directing the interview is one which must be learned. It is, however, one of the more difficult techniques for the nurse to use comfortably. If she is uncomfortable with the silence, her anxiety will be communicated to the patient, causing him to feel that the interview must be a steady stream of conversation or that something is wrong if any pause occurs. She must strive to overcome the tendency to hastily terminate all silences. If the nurse can learn to be comfortable with these pauses in the interview, the patient will usually end the silence, often with pertinent and useful information. Up to a point, the tension produced by the silence can be a force which will encourage the patient to talk.

According to Richardson and associates, a short silence terminated by the respondent is likely to produce a relatively lengthly response. This occurs for a number of reasons:

1. The patient may have needed a short pause in order to formulate his thoughts before continuing to speak
2. The patient may have interpreted the silence as meaning that the interviewer wanted him to continue speaking along the same lines
3. The patient may have found the silence uncomfortable and continued to talk just to end the silence.[43]

The nurse must learn to evaluate the patient's ability to tolerate any tension produced by silence. She can usually tell from the patient's nonverbal behavior whether the silence is being purposefully utilized, or if he is waiting for her to say something. When the patient shows signs of becoming increasingly uncomfortable the nurse should take measures to terminate the silence. For example:

"You were saying that you feel uncomfortable asking anyone to help you."
"Is there anything else?"
"Can you tell me more about what happens when you become angry?"
"What are you thinking about now?"

If the patient stops speaking in the middle of a topic, the nurse can encourage him to continue by merely saying "And?" or "Then?" She may also repeat the last few words of the patient's last sentence, thus indicating that she expects him to continue talking. For example, "Your worries keep you awake. . . ."

Blocks to Effective Interviewing

Effective interviewing requires the ability to make the patient comfortable with the interviewer and the interview situation, to ask questions which are planned to obtain the necessary information, to listen attentively, and to respond in ways which tell the patient that the nurse is listening and which encourage him to talk. The procedures discussed below inhibit communication and are included here to familiarize the nurse with these obstacles in order that she may be better able to establish effective nurse-patient interaction.

Value judgments. Making value judgments or moralizing statements may cause the patient to withhold information. He may refrain from further discussion rather than risk disapproval from the nurse. Therefore, the nurse must convey an attitude that is nonmoralistic and nonjudgmental; she must not impose her own biases, reactions, and values. For example, if the patient says he hates hospitals, the nurse's response should not be "It's wrong to feel that way" (value judgment), but rather "What are some of the things that make you feel that way?"

False or inappropriate reassurance. Making comments which give false or inappropriate reassurance may keep the patient from expressing his thoughts or feelings. For example, if the patient expresses concern about his upcoming operation, the nurse should not reply "Don't worry. Everything will be fine." Instead, she should say "What are some of the things concerning the operation which upset you?"

Advice and opinions. Offering advice or opinions inhibits the patient from exploring his own ideas, thoughts, and feelings related to his problems. There are times when the patient will ask the nurse for her opinions or advice. She should attempt to have him express his own opinions and/or make his own decision about the problem. Even when they request it, most people do not really want advice or opinions, but rather someone to listen

54

to them so that they can arrive at their own decisions. By giving the patient the information he needs in order to make his own judgments or reach a realistic solution to his problems, the nurse can avoid stating her opinion about the matter or advising the patient about what she thinks he should do. Another alternative is to direct questions, ideas, and feelings back to the patient and encourage him to make his own decision. For example, to the patient who asks "Do you think I should have surgery?" the nurse may reply "What are your thoughts about the matter?"[44]

Leading questions. A leading question is one which: 1) makes it easier or more tempting for the patient to give one answer rather than another, 2) uses words which are emotionally loaded so as to evoke one response rather than another, and/or 3) encourages a particular response by associating one of the alternative responses with a goal so desirable that it can scarcely be denied.[45,46]

Many patients have difficulty contradicting the nurse. If the nurse's question implies that a particular answer is expected, the patient will usually choose that answer rather than offend her or risk her disapproval. Florence Nightingale wrote that, "Patients are completely taken aback by . . . leading questions, and give only the exact amount of information asked for, even when they know it to be completely misleading. The shyness of the patient is seldom allowed for. . . . leading questions always collect inaccurate information."[47] Some examples of alternatives to the various types of leading questions are: "How do you feel now?" rather than "You feel better now, don't you?"; "What are some of your thoughts when you are caring for your baby?" rather than "Would you say that you enjoy caring for your baby?"; and "Have you felt any dizziness or faintness this morning?" rather than "You know the doctor said you could go home as soon as you stopped having dizzy spells. Have you had any today?"

"Why" questions. To answer a "why" question the patient must understand the reasons underlying his thoughts, feelings, and behavior. If he does not possess this insight, he will usually: 1) give partial answers or superficial reasons, 2) invent causes just to please the nurse, or 3) avoid answering the why.[48] Peplau states that the why question usually has an intimidating effect because it asks for reasons which the patient is not likely to know.[49] If the patient knew why he was uncomfortable or why he wasn't sleeping, he would probably be able to deal with the situation. In order to discover the reason, it is more effective to ask questions which require the patient to describe what happens when he is uncomfortable or can't sleep. For example, instead of asking "Why can't you sleep?" the nurse should ask "What happens that seems to keep you awake?" or "What do you think about while you are awake?" These responses encourage the patient to describe the difficulty without asking him to give an explanation for it. Much valuable information can be obtained in this manner without asking "why?" Questions asking "what?" or "how?" call for a description rather than a reason.

TERMINATION OF THE INTERVIEW

It is important that the interview be drawn to a definite close and not be left "hanging in mid-air" with the patient feeling that nothing has been accomplished during the particular interaction.[50] Techniques for terminating interviews should be preplanned, friendly, help the patient to feel that he cooperated with the nurse by giving her the information she needed, and give him an idea of what he may expect next. It is the nurse's responsibility to plan and implement a termination that meets these criteria. Several techniques are discussed in this section.

Statement by the nurse that she has the information she needs to begin planning the patient's nursing care. At this time the nurse may ask the patient if there is anything else he would like to tell her that would help the nursing staff plan his nursing care. Sometimes ordinary courtesy will be sufficient to terminate the interview, such as, "Thank you for talking with me. I have the information I need to begin planning your nursing care." If she has the time, the nurse may also remark that, "I've had my chance to ask you questions. Perhaps you have questions you would like to ask me."

Reference to predetermined time limits. It is important that the nurse tell the patient at the beginning of the interview the approximate length of time she will be with him. When the time limit has been set beforehand, it is easier for the nurse to bring the interview to an end by referring to the time limit originally set. When the nurse has almost finished the interview she may say, "I only have a few more questions to ask you." or "We'll be finished in five or ten minutes."

Terminal summarization. Terminal summarization is a method of coordinating what the nurse and patient have discussed during the interview. When the nurse has obtained the information she needs, she may end the interview by summarizing some of the pertinent data elicited from the patient. She may ask the patient to verify the accuracy of the summary and make any necessary corrections. The nurse may also use this technique by summarizing the needs and problems identified by the patient. For example, the nurse may say, "From what you've told me, you have difficulty falling asleep, getting out of bed by yourself, and walking without a walker. You'd like an extra pillow and a talk with your doctor. I'll get you a pillow now and I'll come back later and discuss plans to help you with your sleeping and walking, getting you out of bed, and about seeing your doctor."

Reference to the future. Referring to the future leads the way for planning subsequent meetings with the patient. The nurse needs to tell the patient whether or not she plans to see him again, and for how long (throughout his hospitalization, while he is on the particular unit, and so on). When at all possible, the nurse tells the patient the day and time she will return and for what purpose. Letting the patient know what to expect in the future, what the nurse intends to do, and what she wants the patient to do, helps end the interview on a positive note. For example, the nurse may say, "I have the information I need to begin planning what we need to do for you. I am going to go think about these plans now and will be back about 3:30 to talk with you about them."

Giving the patient something to think about until the next interaction can also be an effective termination technique. For example, the nurse may say, "You said that you had questions about the tests the doctor said you'd have. Between now and when I see you tomorrow, I'd like you to think about and write down your questions and then we'll talk about them." The nurse may also refer to topics which the patient seemed to want to discuss, but which she either excluded or curtailed because of her time limit. The nurse may say, "You were telling me about your sons when we had to go on with the questions I had. I'd enjoy hearing more about what you were saying. If you'd like to, we can talk about that when I see you tomorrow."

RECORDING THE DATA

The Nursing History must be recorded at the time it is taken. This not only saves time but is necessary to obtain a complete, detailed, and accurate data base from which to work. Miller and associates note that research on interviewing technique has shown that ". . . at best only one-third of the pertinent responses in an interview are recorded by recall immediately after the interviewee has gone."[51]

The nurse should explain to the patient at the beginning of the interview that she will be writing the information she learns from him. Patients do not usually mind this as long as they feel that the interviewer is listening to them. They appreciate it as an effort to be as complete and accurate as possible. Many beginners have difficulty listening to the patient, summarizing what has been said and then writing. They attempt to write every word the patient says. Not only is this not possible, it is not useful. It cannot be emphasized enough that the nurse needs to:

1. Listen to the patient's answer
2. Summarize the pertinent information
3. *Then* write the data.

Note: Refer to Chapter 3 for the guidelines for recording data in the Nursing History.

SUMMARY

The nurse must use imagination to find ways to obtain the information she needs. While there is no set of rules which will guarantee successful interviewing, there are some general guidelines which may help the interviewer obtain the needed information, avoid mistakes, learn how to conserve her efforts, and establish and maintain effective interpersonal relationships with patients. Each nurse must determine which techniques work best for her and familiarize herself with various alternative techniques for use as circumstances demand. The development of skills in the area of data collection is necessary for effective nursing care.

REFERENCES

1. Stevenson, Ian: *Medical History-Taking.* Harper and Row, New York, 1960, p. vii.
2. Beveridge, W. I. B.: *The Art of Scientific Investigation,* third edition. W. W. Norton and Company, Inc., New York, 1957, p. 101.
3. Smith, Henry Clay: *Sensitivity to People.* McGraw-Hill Book Company, New York, 1966, pp. 113, 114.
4. Beveridge, op. cit., p. 102.
5. Mumford, Emily, and Skipper, James K.: *Sociology in Hospital Care.* Harper and Row, Publishers, New York, 1967, pp. 76, 77.
6. Ibid., p. 72.
7. Kahn, Robert L., and Cannell, Charles F.: *The Dynamics of Interviewing.* John Wiley and Sons, Inc., New York, 1957, p. 16.
8. Bingham, Walter Van Dyke, and Moore, Bruce Victor: *How to Interview,* fourth revised edition. Harper and Row, Publishers, New York, 1959, p. 63.
9. Marshall, Jon C., and Feeney, Sally: "Structured versus intuitive intake interview." *Nursing Research* 21:272, 1972.
10. Kahn and Cannell, op. cit., p. 209.
11. Ibid., p. 18.
12. Ibid., p. 19.
13. Bingham and Moore, op. cit., p. 63.
14. Vanderzanden, James W., and Vanderzanden, Marion V.: "The interview—What questions should the nurse ask and how should she ask them?" *Nursing Outlook* 11:743, 1963.
15. Fenlason, Anne F.: *Essentials in Interviewing.* Harper and Row, Publishers, New York, 1952, p. 123.
16. Kahn and Cannell, op. cit., p. 92.
17. Ibid., p. 107.
18. Ibid., p. 108.
19. Brammer, Lawrence M., and Shostrom, Everett L.: *Therapeutic Psychology: Fundamentals of Counseling and Psychotherapy.* Prentice-Hall, Inc., Englewood Cliffs, 1960, p. 171.
20. Bingham and Moore, op. cit., p. 146.
21. Kahn and Cannell, op. cit., pp. 80, 81.
22. Vanderzanden and Vanderzanden, op. cit., p. 744.
23. Kahn and Cannell, op. cit., p. 162.
24. Vanderzanden and Vanderzanden, op. cit., p. 743.
25. Greenhill, Maurice H.: "Interviewing with a purpose." *American Journal of Nursing* 56:1260, 1956.
26. Benjamin, Alfred: *The Helping Interview.* Houghton Mifflin Company, Boston, 1969, p. 111.
27. Greenhill, op. cit., p. 1261.
28. Richardson, Stephan A., Dohrenwend, Barbara Snell, and Klein, David: *Interviewing: Its Forms and Functions.* Basic Books, Inc., New York, 1965, pp. 198, 199.
29. Durr, Carol A.: "Hands that help . . . but how?" *Nursing Forum* X:398, 1971.
30. Richardson, Dohrenwend, and Klein, op. cit., p. 222.
31. Kahn and Cannell, op. cit., pp. 107, 108.
32. Ibid., p. 206.
33. Hays, Joyce Samhammer, and Larson, Kenneth H.: *Interacting with Patients.* The Macmillan Company, New York, 1963, p. 15.
34. Kahn and Cannell op. cit., p. 208.
35. Travelbee, Joyce: *Interpersonal Aspects of Nursing.* F. A. Davis Company, Philadelphia, 1966, p. 108.

58

36. Brammer and Shostrom, op. cit., p. 177.
37. Ibid., pp. 179, 180.
38. Ibid., p. 175.
39. Benjamin, op. cit., p. 118.
40. Richardson, Dohrenwend, and Klein, op. cit., p. 163.
41. Hays and Larson, op. cit., p. 19.
42. Richardson, Dohrenwend, and Klein, op. cit., pp. 164, 165.
43. Ibid., p. 204.
44. Hays, Joyce Samhammer: "Analysis of Nurse-Patient Communications." *Nursing Outlook* 14:34, 1966.
45. Bingham and Moore, op. cit., p. 74.
46. Kahn and Cannell, op. cit., pp. 127, 128.
47. Nightingale, Florence: *Notes on Nursing: What It Is and What It Is Not.* Harrison and Sons, London, 1859, p. 61.
48. Hays, op. cit., p. 32.
49. Peplau, Hildegard E.: "Talking with patients." *American Journal of Nursing* 60:965, 1960.
50. Brammer and Shostrom, op. cit., p. 201.
51. Miller, George E., et al.: *Teaching and Learning in Medical School.* Harvard University Press, Cambridge, 1961, p. 265.

SECTION TWO

Application

5

THE PROCESS OF CLINICAL THINKING

The first section of this text introduced a particular system of nursing practice, the rationale for the development of the Clinical Nursing Tool, and the purposes for which it may be used. Discussion of the problem-oriented system and the scientific method specifically emphasized the first phase of each, the collection of data. The role of the Nursing History, Part A of the Clinical Nursing Tool, as a defined data base was explained, and guidelines and techniques for its collection were provided. Now it is time to proceed with the remaining stages of the scientific method and the problem-oriented system, referred to as the "process of clinical thinking" or Part B of the Clinical Nursing Tool. This involves: 1) the problem list, 2) the initial plan, including nursing care objectives and nursing orders, 3) evaluation and modification of the plan through problem-related progress notes, and 4) the discharge, transfer, or expiration note.

This process is a scientific approach to clinical problem solving. Its method of planning and evaluating nursing care clearly demonstrates the thought process, judgment, and creativity of the nurse. By providing a written record of the nurse's contribution, it enables measurement of the effects of nursing care.

Clinical problem solving requires the ability to select relevant data, and to manipulate, interpret, analyze, synthesize, and evaluate information. The conversion of raw data into a meaningful problem list necessitates disciplined thought. The ability to make sound judgments in formulating a plan of management for solving these problems demands cognitive skills of the highest order.[1] The acquisition and utilization of these skills have been variously termed "critical thinking," "reflective thinking," and "problem solving." In essence, these mental skills are techniques for defining and managing problems.

The "Cognitive Domain" of the *Taxonomy of Educational Objectives* outlines a hierarchy of intellectual skills and abilities involved in the problem-solving process.[2] The first category is the recall and recognition of knowledge. Next are the intellectual abilities arranged in ascending order: comprehension, application, analysis, synthesis, and evaluation. Each classification within the hierarchy demands the use of skills from the previous (lower) classifications. The brief outline which follows gives the reader an idea of what is involved in the utilization of these cognitive skills. No attempt is made to reproduce the excellent explanations and examples included in the taxonomy. For these, the reader is referred to the original source.

The knowledge category of the taxonomy is divided into three main subcategories:

1. Knowledge of specific information
   a. Terminology
   b. Facts
2. Knowledge of ways and means of dealing with specifics
   a. Methods of inquiry, including techniques and procedures employed to investigate particular problems and phenomena
   b. Ways of treating and presenting ideas and phenomena, including organizing, studying, judging, and criticizing
   c. Classification and categories regarded as fundamental for a given subject field or problem
   d. Trends and sequences of phenomena
   e. Criteria by which principles, opinions, and behavior are tested or judged
3. Knowledge of the universals and abstractions in a field
   a. Principles and generalizations (abstractions) which summarize observations and are of value in explaining, describing, predicting, or determining the most appropriate and relevant action or direction to be taken
   b. Theories and structures which show the interrelationships and organization of a great range of facts

The hierarchy includes those cognitive components involved in clinical problem solving:

1. Comprehension
   a. Translation
   b. Interpretation
   c. Extrapolation
2. Application
   a. Use of abstractions in specific and concrete situations
3. Analysis
   a. Analysis of elements: identification of the parts of a communication
   b. Analysis of relationships: the interaction or connection between parts of a communication

64

    c. Analysis of organizational principles: the arrangement and structure which hold together the communication as a whole
4. Synthesis

    Synthesis involves the putting together of pieces of information, that is, arranging or combining the parts in such a way as to constitute a pattern or structure not clearly there before.[3] This may include:

    a. Production of a unique communication to convey ideas, feelings, and/or experiences to others

    b. Production of a plan or proposed set of operations to be carried out

    c. Development of a set of abstract relations to classify or explain certain data on phenomena

5. Evaluation

    Evaluation is ". . . the making of judgments about the value, for some purpose, of ideas, works, solutions, methods, material, etc. It involves the use of criteria as well as standards for appraising the extent to which particulars are accurate, effective, economical, or satisfying."[4] While the judgments may be either quantitative or qualitative, they must be based on criteria, not opinion.

    a. Judgments may be made in terms of internal evidence: logical accuracy and consistency

    b. Judgments may be made in terms of external criteria: ends (goals) to be satisfied, rules or standards

In summary, just as manual procedures must be practiced for the nurse to become adept in their performance, the cognitive skills must also be consistently exercised and evaluated to achieve proficiency. This requires careful, thorough auditing of the thought process using the problem-oriented patient records employed in this system of nursing practice.

There is often a breakdown in the nursing process after the initial collection of facts (the Nursing History), or in some instances after the problem list. Perhaps one reason for this noncompletion is the lack of opportunities in schools of nursing and health agencies to practice the cognitive skills as outlined in Bloom's taxonomy. However, it is felt that if the nurse has access to the steps of the process (the Clinical Nursing Tool) and information pertaining to the performance of each step, she will try to complete it to the best of her ability. The following chapters include information helpful in understanding the thinking process involved with identification and management of nursing problems, and evaluation of progress toward their resolution. In addition, directions are given for writing the problem list, the plan of care (including the writing of nursing care objectives and nursing orders), the progress notes, and the discharge, transfer or expiration note.

REFERENCES

1.   Chambers, Wilda: "Nursing diagnosis." *American Journal of Nursing* 62:102–104, 1962.

2.   Bloom, Benjamin S. (ed.): *Taxonomy of Educational Objectives: The Classification of Educational Goals, Handbook I: The Cognitive Domain*. David McKay Company, Inc., New York, 1956..
3.   Ibid., p. 162.
4.   Ibid., p. 185.

6

THE PROBLEM LIST

The patient's nursing problems must be explicitly defined before the subsequent steps of the problem-solving process can be initiated for their systematic management. Therefore, the nurse must first make a thorough assessment of all available data, including the Nursing History, medical history, medical plan of care, laboratory reports, and any information contributed by family, friends, or the other members of the health team. This assessment process consists of analyzing and judging the collected data to identify nursing problems and needs. According to Bower, the nurse must:

1. Extract relevant facts and concepts from the available data
2. Classify and sort these data into groups that demonstrate relationships
3. Make interpretations of the data based on the interrelatedness of these groupings.[1]

RECOGNITION OF PROBLEMS

As stated earlier, a nursing problem is any condition or situation in which a patient requires help to maintain or regain a state of health, or to achieve a peaceful death. It may concern the patient, family, and/or nurse, and may be physiologic, psychologic, sociologic, and/or economic. The problem list is an itemization of nursing problems derived from data collected from and about the patient. Hurst states that the problem list is not simply the identification of the data base by numbers, but that it instead evolves out of the data base.[2] This list serves as an index to the record of nursing care and should thus be kept in the same place in the patient's chart to allow easy reference.

The thought process of the nurse arranges facts into a pattern, leading to the formulation of a nursing diagnosis or problem statement.[3] Nurses have traditionally avoided using the word diagnosis, viewing it as something which only physicians have the right to do. However, *diagnosis* is defined as:

> investigation or analysis of the cause or nature of a condition, situation, or problem; a statement or conclusion about the nature or cause of a phenomenon.[4]

Thus, nurses do, in fact, make diagnoses, whether or not they refer to them as such. The term *nursing diagnosis* may be defined as a conclusion or decision resulting from careful investigation, examination, and analysis of data. However, a nursing diagnosis is limited to those activities which are legally within the province of the professional nurse.

The thought process through which problems are identified or diagnoses are made is influenced by the nurse's background of scientific knowledge, past nursing experiences, and her definition of nursing. For example, using Henderson's definition of nursing (p. 6), the nurse may ask the following questions while examining data in order to identify nursing problems or to make nursing diagnoses.

1. Is there anything with which the patient requires assistance in order to maintain or regain a state of health, or to achieve a peaceful death?
2. Is the reason he needs assistance due to lack of strength, will, and/or knowledge?
3. What kinds of assistance would be most apt to move the patient toward appropriate independence?

Bower states that problems arise when the patient, family, or community

1. Cannot meet a need
2. Needs help to meet a need
3. Is not aware of an unmet need
4. Has a conflict of apparently equally important needs
5. Must choose from several alternative ways of meeting needs.[5]

Thus, a nursing problem exists when the patient lacks the necessary strength, will, and/or knowledge to meet his needs.

In nursing, the terms problem and need are sometimes used incorrectly as synonyms. A need may or may not be a problem. All people have needs but all people do not have nursing problems. The majority of people meet some or all of their own needs without nursing assistance. For example, each person has a basic need to breathe; however, this does not mean that each patient requires nursing assistance to help him meet this need. If patients have the necessary strength, will, and knowledge to provide for their own needs, nursing problems related to these needs will not emerge.

The nurse should not create nursing problems where none exist. The important thing is to make certain that data have been collected and thoroughly examined for problems. When these two steps of the process have been carefully performed, she may decide what assistance is or is not needed. However, this decision must be based on evidence, not assumption, accident, or neglect.

Many of a patient's needs may be met by carrying out the medical plan of care or by "routine" hygienic care. As long as this proves satisfactory, these needs will not present nursing problems and thus will not require a nursing plan of care for their management.

Some problems are obvious (overt) while others are more subtle and not as easily recognized (covert). The nurse may realize that a problem exists, but be unable to specifically define it. In this instance, the problem should be stated at the level of refinement that is known at the time. Usually, through the collection of additional data, the specific problem becomes more obvious and able to be defined. Bower states:

> Overt problems are problems that are easily recognized. Covert problems are problems that are difficult to identify either because of a lack of data, an overlay of other problems, or a lack of objectivity. These problems need to be discovered . . . the nurse needs to gather all available data and employ particular care in systematically sifting out the problem.[6]

RECORDING PROBLEMS

The problem list should include every nursing problem which can be identified from all available data. It evolves through classifying data into particular categories. The data are then analyzed in view of existing knowledge and relationships to other information. The results of this analysis are synthesized into the form of a problem statement. Each problem is listed at the level of refinement that is known and must be defined as explicitly as possible to allow subsequent stages of the problem-solving process to follow in logical sequence. Weed states that question marks and the word "probable" do not belong on the list. Either a problem exists or it does not and, therefore, should be stated in terms which can be supported by data.[7] Bower says that:

> Problem statements need to be clear, simple, complete, and specific. . . . a large part of the solution of a problem lies in knowing what it is you are trying to do.[8]

The statement itself may be expressed in a variety of forms and concern any of several aspects. Durand and Prince state that the nursing diagnosis may be:

1. Descriptive
2. Etiologic
3. Primarily physiologic, primarily psychologic or have both physiologic and psychologic aspects
4. A major medical symptom
5. Anticipated in a certain medical diagnosis
6. Distinct from the medical diagnosis
   a. Due to hospitalization
   b. Due to a complication of the primary illness
7. The same as the medical diagnosis.[9]

Refer to Figure 1 for examples of problem statements.

It is unusual for the nursing problem to be the same as the medical diagnosis. This occurs most often in emergency situations when the nurse's goals and actions are the same as the physician's, or when the available data reveals insufficient information about the effect of the illness on the patient, his knowledge and/or understanding of his illness, and his ability to cope with it. As the specific nursing aspects related to the problem become known, the problem statement should be modified to include this information. For example, if a diabetic patient is admitted to the hospital in a coma, the initial problem statement may be "diabetic coma." However, once the patient is out of coma, the nurse attempts to obtain additional information about the patient, his understanding of his illness, and his usual coping behavior. The data reveals that the patient has not been taking insulin as ordered by his physician because he thought this was necessary only when he began to feel "badly." At this time, the nursing problem would be modified to state "inadequate understanding of insulin administration."

The same nursing problem may be evident in patients having different medical diagnoses since, ". . . the same physiological and psychological processes may be present even when the total patterns as viewed by the physician are different."[10] For example, nausea may be the nursing problem in patients having a medical diagnosis of renal failure, acute appendicitis, or anxiety reaction. Whereas a medical diagnosis serves to summarize a group of signs and symptoms, a nursing problem may state one sign or symptom that focuses on the patient's particular response to his illness. A medical diagnosis often remains the same until the patient recovers or dies. However, since assessment is a continuous process the nurse's problem statement usually is not static but must be altered as the condition of the patient indicates and as more information is collected, analyzed, and validated.

When the problem is modified, the original problem list is amended accordingly. Revision of the problem list may occur at any time. This modification is not accomplished by erasure but rather the insertion of the word "modified," followed by the new statement of the problem. In the instance where the problem is resolved, the term "resolved" is written

Descriptive	1. Cries when mentions loss of job and appearance 2. Atrophy of adipose tissue on anterior of upper thighs 3. Nervous when with people 4. Must have orange juice and hot coffee q.d. to maintain bowel pattern
Etiological	1. Weakness due to lack of activity 2. Hyperventilates when nervous 3. Atrophy of adipose tissue from failure to rotate injection sites
Primarily physiological Primarily psychological Having aspects of both	1. Dry skin 2. Nervous and fear of dying 3. Obesity or insomnia or nausea
Major medical symptom	1. Weakness 2. Headache 3. Pain 4. Nausea 5. Dehydration
Anticipated in a certain medical condition	1. Tendency to bleed (with inadequate platelets) 2. Pain (with surgery) 3. Dehydration (with diarrhea and vomiting)
Distinct from the medical diagnosis or condition	1. Worried about paying bills 2. Toothache 3. Generalized skin rash
Medical diagnosis	1. Diabetic coma

FIGURE 1

following the problem to which it pertains. Each change should be dated in the appropriate space on the problem list (see Fig. 2). This date should correspond with the date of the progress note in which the data clarifying the problem or indicating its resolution is recorded. By updating the problem list in this manner, a record of all revisions is maintained and the thought process of the nurse preserved (see Fig. 3).

Collection of additional information may reveal that problems which were first seen as separate are actually related. When problems are combined, use the number of the first problem for the combined problem statement. For example, if Problem 2 "approved for kidney transplant

#	Nursing Problems	Date	
		First Noted or Change of Title	Resolved
1			
2			
3			
4			
5			
6			
7			
8			

FIGURE 2

program" and Problem 3 "feels nervous" combine to become "fear of surgery," this now becomes Problem 2. The two previous problem statements are discontinued as active problems by placing the date of this change in the appropriate column (see Fig. 4).

When several nursing problems are related to one major problem, the major problem may be listed and subdivided to manage the various manifestations. This frequently occurs with a medical problem involving two or more nursing problems. If in doubt about whether or not problems are

#	Nursing Problems	Date	
		First Noted or Change of Title	Resolved
1	Atrophy of adipose tissue on anterior upper thighs -- Modified -- Atrophy of adipose tissue from failure to rotate injection sites	3-14-73 3-15-73	
2	Weakness -- Modified -- Weakness from lack of exercise -- Resolved	3-14-73 3-16-73	 3-20-73
3	Nausea -- Resolved	3-14-73	3-16-73

FIGURE 3

related, list separately those problems requiring individual management (see Fig. 5).

Weed speaks of the problem-oriented system as one in which all members of the health team use one problem list. However, this is not the case in many institutions. While this text is written as though nurses' notes are separate from physicians', the information and directions also apply to the situation Weed advocates. When one problem list is used by medical and nursing staff, anyone can add a new problem to the list provided an adequate definition of it is recorded in a progress note.

Nelson states that a "complete" problem list can be overwhelming if it is assumed that a single individual must solve every problem noted. He points out that no individual can ever deal with all types of problems, but that he may be able to get help to solve a problem—*if* it is recognized on the problem list.[11] For example, Mrs. P. came to the hospital with ascites and pitting edema of the feet and legs, and was admitted to find the cause of these problems. Her primary concern, however, was to have her five remaining teeth extracted. Through recognizing the problem, writing it on the problem list and bringing it to the attention of the physician in the form of a request for a dental referral, this problem was solved through the help

#	Nursing Problems	Date	
		First Noted or Change of Title	Resolved
1	Reduced kidney function a. Nausea	3-14-73 3-17-73	
2	Approved for kidney transplant program -- Modified -- Fear of surgery	3-14-73 3-16-73	
3	Feels nervous -- See #2	3-14-73	3-16-73
4	Nausea -- See #1	3-14-73	3-17-73

FIGURE 4

of others (the physician who made the referral and the dentist who pulled the teeth). It is unlikely that this problem would have been resolved had it not been recognized by the nurse as a problem.

Nelson further states that there is no requirement that every problem on the list be solved. However, a complete list aids in setting priorities, keeping problems and plans in context, identifying relationships among problems, and managing the complete patient. Dr. Weed states, "Multiple problems may interact, and sophisticated understanding and management of any one of them requires at least an awareness of all of them."[12]

In instances when it is not possible to collect all the information required by the defined data base, Problem #1 on the problem list should be "incomplete data base." Other problems which can be identified from the available data are listed and dated accordingly. When the defined data base has been recorded, Problem # 1 is resolved and the date entered on the list (see Fig. 6).

The problem list should be shared with the patient. It is essential that the nurse determine whether or not the patient agrees with the problem as stated and whether there is anything else he would like to add. This communicates to the patient the nurse's understanding of his problems and gives him an idea of what to expect regarding his nursing care.

Randall identifies errors commonly made in formulating the complete

#	Nursing Problems	Date	
		First Noted or Change of Title	Resolved
1	Joint pain a. Pain in all joints b. Limited range of motion c. Unable to walk s̄ assistance	3-16-73 3-16-73 3-16-73 3-16-73	
2	Feels depressed	3-16-73	
3	Reduced kidney function a. Nausea b. Diarrhea c. Failure to adhere to fluid restriction d. Weakness	3-20-73 3-20-73 3-20-73 3-22-73 3-23-73	
4	Control of Diabetes Mellitus a. Inadequate understanding of insulin administration	3-20-73 3-21-73	

FIGURE 5

problem list.[13] The mistakes he identifies are discussed in relation to the physician; however, they are equally appropriate for nurses, and examples related to nursing problems have been added.

1. Failure to list problems noted in the data base. This may be due to:
    a. Overlooking the significance of a finding.
        Example: Failure to list "sores in mouth" as a problem. If the sores are not considered significant, the possibility that the patient is not eating because of a sore mouth may be overlooked.
    b. Attributing an abnormality to another problem.
        Example: The discovery of skin breakdown in a patient on bed rest could mistakenly be assumed to be due to immobility when in fact it might indicate inadequate nutritional intake and insufficient protein.

#	Nursing Problems	Date	
		First Noted or Change of Title	Resolved
1	Incomplete data base	3-14-73	3-15-73
2	Nausea	3-14-73	
3	Back pain	3-15-73	
4	Worried about finances	3-15-73	
5	Fear of inability to care for self	3-15-73	

FIGURE 6

2. Construction of a cumbersome problem list. This is usually due to:
   a. Failure to synthesize data.
      Example: The data base reveals the following information. The patient never feels hungry, fills up after "a few bites," eats two meals daily, eats less when upset, has no energy, and has lost 30 pounds in the past six months. Rather than stating the above information as separate problems, this data could be synthesized into one problem statement, such as "anorexia."
   b. Use of data base on the problem list.
      Example: The problem list should not merely repeat information found in the data base, it should determine problems based on this information. Thus, rather than stating one problem as "skin breakdown on sacrum," list four separate problems as:
      1. Bed rest order
      2. Not eating
      3. Does not voluntarily change positions
      4. Incontinent of urine and stool.

c. Addition of temporary problems to the list rather than handling them within the progress notes.

   Example: If the patient develops a headache at some point during his hospitalization, this may be recorded in the progress notes as additional data along with what is done to relieve the headache or to make the patient more comfortable. An evaluation of the effectiveness of the nursing actions is included along with any future plans if indicated. Such a problem does not need to be added to the problem list. However, the problem could be added to the problem list should it become persistent.

3. Including guesses of probabilities on the problem list rather than stating the problem at the level of refinement supported by the available data.

   Example: Available data shows that the patient is frequently found crying and that she is scheduled for surgery in two days. Writing on the problem list "probable fear of surgery" is an inclusion of a guess or probability on the problem list. The patient could be crying for a variety of reasons and these reasons must be determined, not assumed, by the nurse. The problem should be stated simply as "cries frequently" until the data allows a more specific definition of the problem.

4. Attributing new problems to old problems.

   Example: Attributing failure to eat to a previous problem of anorexia when in fact it is due to an inability to feed oneself because of a painful phlebitis in the arm.

5. Failure to update the list after new data are collected defeats the purpose of the list and may lead to confusion and mismangement. This is shown by:

   a. Failure to differentiate an active problem from one which has been resolved.

      Example: Leaving "weakness" as an active problem on the list after objective data indicate that the patient is able to walk a predetermined distance steadily and without assistance and the subjective data reveal that the patient no longer feels weak.

   b. Failure to add new problems to the list.

      Example: This is self-evident; however, if during hospitalization the patient develops a phlebitis, this should be added to the problem list.

   c. Failure to reverse a cumbersome or inaccurate problem list. If subsequent data indicate a relationship between what were first listed as separate problems, these problems may be combined into one problem statement thus eliminating the necessity of dealing separately with each problem while not interfering with the accuracy of the past record.

77

Example:
#1 anorexia—See #5
#2 insomnia—See #5
#3 loss of job—See #5
#4 tired—See #5
#5 depression

6. Failure to date accurately all entries on the problem list. This makes reliable auditing of the record difficult if not impossible.

SUMMARY

Each patient should have a complete problem list which reveals his nursing problems as defined from data derived from the Nursing History, family, and other members of the health team. The problem list is not static, but is updated as new data become available. It aids in focusing on particular problems and identifying relationships that might not be evident otherwise. Once the problem list has been established, all subsequent plans, including nursing care objectives, orders, and progress notes are recorded using the number of the problem statement to which they specifically relate. Directions for the formulation and use of the problem list are reviewed below.

DIRECTIONS FOR WRITING THE PROBLEM LIST

1. Title the sheet of paper "Problem List."
2. Place the problem list in the patient's chart following the Nursing History or in another consistent place. The problem list serves as an index to the record of nursing care.
3. Number each entry on the problem list.
4. Date each entry on the problem list.
5. State all of the patient's nursing problems—physiologic, psychologic, sociologic, and/or economic.
6. State each problem at the level of refinement known at the time it is entered on the problem list, and which can be supported by recorded data. The problem title should indicate exactly what is known, omitting guesses or probabilities. The list should present evidence that the nurse understands the patient's disease and related components.
7. State the problem so that it reflects the task of the nurse or communicates an aim or direction. For example, write "inadequate understanding of insulin administration" rather than "insulin administration."
8. The statement of the problem may be expressed in a variety of forms: a) descriptive, b) etiologic, c) primarily physiologic, primarily psychologic, or have both physiologic and psychologic aspects, d) a major medical symptom, e) anticipated in a certain medical diagnosis, f) distinct from the medical diagnosis, or g) the same as the medical diagnosis.

9. The problem may require:
   a. The collection of additional data
   b. Nursing intervention:
      1. Maintenance of usual patterns. This requires recognition of usual patterns with which the patient requires assistance.
      2. Treatment of presenting problems.
      3. Prevention of complications.
   c. Giving information to patient, family, or other members of the health team.

10. Include those problems which concern the patient's family or other significant people as well as those which primarily involve the patient.

11. List as an entity several signs and symptoms or facts that go together when it is *certain* that they belong together.

12. If in doubt about whether or not problems are related, list separately those problems requiring individual management.

13. Keep the problem list current. It should accurately reflect the patient's status at all times, thus necessitating continuous evaluation. The list is updated:
   a. When a new problem is identified
   b. When a problem is resolved
   c. When a problem is clarified thus necessitating a new title
   d. When two or more problems are combined.
The date recorded for the addition, deletion, or modification of problems should correspond with the date of the progress note containing the data upon which this decision is based.

14. Revise the problem statement by inserting the term "modified" followed by the new statement of the problem. Record the date.

15. If problems are combined, use the number of the first problem of the group and date the subsequent problems in the "resolved" column thus indicating what has been done.

16. If several nursing problems are related to one major problem, but require different management, list the major problem and enter the related ones as subdivisions of it.

17. If a problem is resolved, write the word "resolved" following the problem statement and enter the date in the appropriate column.

18. When a new problem is identified, number it, add it to the list, and record the date.

19. When the complete data base has not been collected, record Problem #1 as "incomplete data base." When it has been obtained, write "resolved" and enter the date.

20. Review the problem list with the patient.

21. Once the problem list is established, record all subsequent plans and data in the progress notes under the numbered and titled problem to which they specifically relate.

NURSING HISTORY AND PROBLEM LIST

The following example demonstrates a Nursing History and the initial problem list formulated from this particular data base. As with the previous example, all identifying information has been eliminated or changed.

Addressograph
Stamp

Nursing History

1-10-73 (1000)

I. Vital statistics: Second General Hospital admission for Leila Hart, a 36 year old married woman from Peabody, Fl.

II. Patient's understanding of illness: Came to hospital because of lupus, "a disease that means you are allergic to the sun." Says lupus keeps the red blood count down and causes damage to liver and kidneys. Believes illness to be caused by being left in sun for an hour waiting for ambulance following car accident. Has been "up and down" since onset of illness; hasn't felt like eating, can't work or care for children (older daughter has had to stay home from school to care for mother and younger children), "nerves" have been "bad" (feels shaky and cries). Illness has caused pain, skin problems, loss of hair.

III. Patient's expectations: Doesn't know what will happen while she's in hospital. Says can't get rid of lupus but that it will go away after a while and come back again. Wants to be able to walk and care for herself. Expects nurses to help her onto bed pan and to talk c̄ her.

IV. Brief social and cultural history: Hasn't worked since onset of illness 1 year ago; used to work as maid in motel. Completed 11th grade. Family members include husband, 4 children (ages 15, 11, 10, 8); lives c̄ same. Older daughter most significant person. Concerned about daughter missing school when patient home ill (daughter back in school now).

V. Significant data in terms of:
   A. Sleeping patterns: Retires 2100; arises 0630. Washes face, brushes teeth, and watches TV ā bed. No difficulty falling asleep; does not wake up during the night. Uses 2 pillows, 1 under head and 1 under feet to "lift and keep them from hurting so."
   B. Eliminating patterns: B.M. q.o.d. p̄ cup of coffee. Last B.M. 1-9-73. Coffee usually maintains pattern. Gets constipated

(tightness in stomach) once/week. Takes Exlax to relieve difficulty. No problem c̄ voiding.

C. Breathing: states has no problems breathing. At present nose breathing, using thoracic muscles, breathing inaudible c̄ no signs of distress.

D. Eating and drinking patterns: Breakfast (0900): coffee, egg, bread, orange juice; Lunch (1200): hamburger, mashed potatoes, soda; Dinner (1800): meat, rice, beans, coffee or soda. Drinks 8 glasses fluid/day consisting of water, juice, cocoa, soda, coffee; prefers water and cocoa. Dislikes food s̄ salt. No medical (at this time) or religious restrictions. No difficulty c̄ nausea, vomiting, chewing, swallowing. Needs help cutting food and opening containers due to pain in joints. Hasn't felt like eating, "just not hungry." Nothing seems to help appetite.

E. Skin integrity: Skin is black c̄ light blotches over arms, legs, face and is tight, rough, scaly, and dry. Decubitus ulcer on sacral area 3″ in diameter, ¼″ deep. Area clean, not draining. Skin particularly scaly on feet, forearms, lower legs, face. Mucous membranes of mouth dry, not broken. Lips dry, cracked. Cares for skin c̄ Ivory soap and lotion "all over body" for dry skin. Tub bath q.o.d. anytime before 1100 (ā soap opera). Washes face when gets up. Wears no makeup. Brushes teeth q.d. p̄ breakfast. Has lost patches of hair; remaining hair scant. Unable to bathe self due to limited and painful movement of joints. Says she needs someone to bathe her.

F. Activity: Patient on bedrest; walking not observed but patient says she's unable to walk due to weakness and painful joints. Observed full R.O.M. in neck and arms at shoulder and elbow; wrists and fingers painful c̄ any movement. With assistance, legs can be flexed at hip, abducted and adducted s̄ pain. Able to extend legs; flexion of knees limited to 20°; pain c̄ any attempt to move feet. Reports feeling weak, makes it hard to even move parts that do not hurt. With weakness and pain in joints, cannot cut food, open containers, bathe self. No prostheses.

G. Recreation: Listens to record player, watches TV.

H. Interpersonal and communicative patterns: Likes to talk c̄ people and feels comfortable once gets to know others. Gets "nervous," uncomfortable c̄ people she doesn't know. Begins to feel at ease if others sit down and talk c̄ her. Nonverbal behavior; lying on back, keeps still ("hurts to move"), licks lips. Verbal behavior: answers questions, volunteers information, does not ask questions or change subject, speaks clearly.

I. Temperament: Gets irritated when children won't listen to her or daughter. Arguing upsets patient. Says feels nervous (shaky) when upset or irritated. Tells others what bothers her.

J. Dependency and independency patterns: Unable to help others now. Used to take food to neighbors when sick and care for children when neighbor went shopping. Others help patient by cooking, helping c̄ housework, taking her to clinic, looking in to see how she's doing. Plans how to spend money c̄ husband so can get what they want. Asks when wants something. Feels comfortable asking for help unless others fuss when she asks; then stops asking and tries to do for herself. Likes to do what can for self; upset c̄ weakness and inability to feed and bathe self.

K. Senses: Wears glasses for reading; no other problems c̄ sight. No problems hearing. Right handed.

L. Menstrual patterns: Menstrual periods occur q. 30 days; 4-day duration. Last menstrual period 1-2-73. No difficulties c̄ menstruation.

VI. Statement of that which helps patient feel cared for: Daughter fixing something special for her to eat and people taking her to see doctor make her feel cared for. Bible and TV are important to patient.

D. Loring, R.N.

#	Nursing Problems	Date First Noted or Change of Title	Resolved
1	Joint pain	1-10-73	
2	Skin breakdown	1-10-73	
3	Mouth dry; lips dry, cracked	1-10-73	
4	Loss of appetite	1-10-73	
5	Feelings related to diminished Functioning	1-10-73	
6	Constipation (potential)	1-10-73	
7	Bible, TV - important items	1-10-73	
8			

REFERENCES

1. Bower, Fay Louise: *The Process of Planning Nursing Care.* The C. V. Mosby Company, St. Louis, 1972, pp. 44–45.
2. Hurst, J. Willis: "How to implement the Weed System: In order to improve patient care, education, and research by improving medical records." *Archives of Internal Medicine* 128:457–458, 1971.
3. Durand, Mary, and Prince, Rosemary: "Nursing diagnosis: Process and decision." *Nursing Forum* V:55, 1966.
4. *Webster's Third New International Dictionary,* G. and C. Merriam Company, Springfield, 1967, p. 622.
5. Bower, op. cit., p. 68.
6. Ibid., p. 12.
7. Weed, Lawrence L.: *Medical Records, Medical Education and Patient Care.*

The Press of Case Western Reserve University, Cleveland, Year Book Medical Publishers, Inc., Chicago, 1969, pp. 39–40.

8. Bower, op. cit., p. 73–74.
9. Durand and Prince, op. cit., pp. 56–57.
10. Ibid., p. 56.
11. Nelson, George E.: "Experiences with the problem-oriented record at the University of Vermont," in Hurst, J. W., and Walker, H. K. (eds.): *The Problem-Oriented System,* MEDCOM, Inc., New York, 1972, pp. 73–74.
12. Weed, op. cit., p. 97.

7

THE INITIAL PLAN

Mager tells the fable of a sea horse who set out to find his fortune. During his journey, he met various sea creatures who sold him different methods of transportation supposed to enable faster travel. Finally, he met a shark who sold him on taking a short cut by way of what was actually the shark's mouth. The sea horse, intent upon completing his trip as quickly as possible, entered the shark's mouth and was devoured. The moral of this fable is that if one is not certain of where he is going, he may arrive someplace else and not even realize what happened.[1]

This chapter concerns the skills involved in formulating the initial plan of nursing care which indicates "where we are going" with the management of a particular patient's nursing care. When we know this, we can evaluate progress toward achieving these objectives and modify the plan of care if necessary. Also discussed are: 1) the parts of the initial plan and their purposes, 2) the various kinds of plans, 3) nursing care objectives and how to write them, 4) nursing orders and how to write them, and 5) the format of the plan and how it may be recorded.

DEFINITION

The *initial plan* refers to *the beginning design, method, or scheme of action by which the patient's nursing problems are to be managed*. It is a statement of the specific methods planned for the solution of each problem identified on the problem list. It is termed *initial* to emphasize that it is a beginning, not a finished product. The plan of care is a continuous process, and as such, is revised whenever new data indicate the need for modification. This chapter concerns only the initial plan. Chapter 8, "The Progress Notes," deals with updating the plan of care since this is where such modification is recorded.

Just as the Nursing History provides the means for organizing data acquired from and about the patient, the initial plan provides the means for utilizing this information to provide the best possible nursing care.

PREPARATION

Factors reflecting consideration of the patient as an individual are recorded in the Nursing History and must be taken into account when formulating the plan of care. Other sources of data to be consulted include: 1) nursing diagnoses, 2) nursing prognosis, 3) nursing care standards, 4) medical diagnoses, 5) medical plan of care, 6) medical prognosis, 7) effect of the disease and treatment regimen (both medical and nursing) on the patient, 8) laboratory reports, 9) problems identified by other members of the health team, 10) plans formulated by them, and 11) literature.

Data from all of the above sources may not be available when the nurse formulates her initial plan since she is often the first person to interview the patient. However, all existing data should be utilized and additional information incorporated into the plan as it becomes available.

RECORDING PROCESS

Each problem on the problem list should have its own plan. The number of the plan should correspond with the number of the problem to which it pertains. Determination of a plan for the solution of each problem includes delineation of nursing care objectives and prescription of nursing orders designed to meet the stated objectives.

The initial plan is recorded following the problem list, dated, and titled "Initial Plan." This phase of the process involves:

1. A discussion of each problem on the problem list
2. An assessment of each problem
3. A plan designed for the management of each problem.

DISCUSSION

This section coordinates all available information pertinent to the problem under examination. Weed states:

> Each problem should be discussed separately. All the available information concerning a given problem should be presented, whether it came from the patient, a relative, a friend, an old chart, a laboratory data book, a pathology slide . . . or the files in an X-ray department. . . .[2]

Discussion of each problem requires use of a knowledge base relevant to the problem at hand and the ability to analyze data for relationships. This is not to imply that the knowledge of all facts must be carried in the head of the nurse at all times. It is meant only to indicate that knowledge of the problem is required for its solution, and seeking knowledge when necessary is essential in any nurse's practice. Thus, literature is a valuable source of information needed to manage nursing problems.

The discussion section of the initial plan is divided into two parts: Subjective data, and objective data.

Subjective data

This consists of information relative to the problem from the patient's point of view. It is that information which the patient reports. Examples of patient statements of subjective data include:

I feel nervous.
I'm afraid of surgery.
My teeth hurt when I chew food.

Objective data

This is the factual information resulting from the nurse's observations pertinent to the given problem. Whenever possible, objective data should reflect quantitative observations or measurements. Examples include:

Size of a decubitus ulcer
Laboratory values
Specific blood pressure readings
Distance walked without evidence of difficulty

Purposes

The discussion of each problem cited in the problem list serves several purposes.
1. It reveals the subjective and objective data which indicated the problem.
2. It provides a baseline against which subsequent observations may be compared and progress measured. For example, if the size of a decubitus ulcer is two inches in diameter, notation of this provides a baseline by which to later determine whether the ulcer is becoming smaller or larger.
3. It reveals the thought process relevant to formulation of plans for management of the problem. For example, if a nursing order for the management of the problem "constipation" states, "Give prune juice q.d. h.s.," the reader may clearly see the data upon which this decision was based—that the patient has a bowel movement only if he drinks prune juice every day at bedtime.
4. It shows the relationship of other problems on the list to the one under consideration. This factor may greatly influence the plans which the nurse prepares. Nursing care objectives and orders which ordinarily would provide satisfactory management of a problem may be contraindicated in view of other problems noted. For example, a nursing order for pushing fluids is

87

an appropriate method for managing the problem of constipation. However, this would be inappropriate when another problem statement indicates that the patient is in congestive heart failure.

It is true that the subjective and objective data recorded in the initial plan are also noted elsewhere in the patient's chart. However, this discussion coordinates all of the relevant factors appearing in different places in the chart, and thus provides more effective utilization of data in planning the patient's nursing care. For example, data pertinent to the problem "constipation" may be found in several sections of category V of the Nursing History: "eliminating patterns"—the usual frequency of bowel elimination, how the patient maintains his pattern, a description of the problem, and what the patient usually does for it; "eating and drinking patterns"—a description of the kinds of foods the patient eats as well as the amount of fluid he drinks daily; "activity"—any related limitation in activity; and "dependency and independency patterns"—the ease with which the patient will ask for help when he needs it. Other data may be found in the patient's Medical History relevant to previous and present bowel problems and treatments. The medical plan of care may reveal plans for a barium enema which could further complicate any problems the patient has with constipation, or orders for medications which are known to be constipating.

ASSESSMENT

This part of the initial plan is a summarization of the nurse's thoughts pertaining to a given problem. It consists of:

1. An analysis of the nature of the problem or a probable explanation for the existence of the problem,
2. The identification of factors which may enhance or inhibit the solution of the problem, such as age, social, cultural, and economic factors, intellectual capacity, the patient's usual ability to cope with stress, and the effects of the patient's illness,
3. An explanation of why the plan will deviate from the usual management of the problem due to conflicts with other interacting problems,
4. The thoughts relative to whether or not nursing intervention should be instituted, and/or
5. A prediction of the probable result of initiating nursing intervention.

It is in this section that the nurse can and should simply state what she thinks. She is free to express her impressions, opinions, and predictions. However, these statements should be based on her knowledge and experiences, and the experiences reported by others in the literature. This is an excellent place to consider available research and statistical information upon which to make a prediction.

Weed makes this statement about the structure of the problem-oriented system:

> When the physician moves within this framework, his ability to choose the important parameters to be followed, his standards of logic, and his sense of responsibility in the attack upon and resolution of the patient's problems can immediately be appreciated.[3]

The framework of the initial plan yields evidence of the nurse's ability to examine problems, see relationships, and choose logical, useful, and scientifically based plans.

THE PLAN

This is the statement of the actual plan for the solution or management of each problem. Specific plans may be categorized as:

1. Plans for collection of additional data to better define a problem or facilitate its management,
2. Plans for dissemination of information pertinent to management of a problem, and/or
3. Plans for the nursing "treatment" of a problem.[4]

Plans for collection of additional data

These plans may be necessary for various reasons:

1. To complete the defined data base
2. To better define the problem
3. To determine the cause of the problem
4. To ascertain the patient's thoughts, feelings, knowledge, goals, and/or questions pertaining to his problem.

Additional data may be collected from many sources. For example, the physician may be asked to explain his thoughts about the patient's medical diagnosis, his prognosis, what he plans to tell the patient about his illness and when he will do this. Information may be obtained from the physical therapist regarding recommendations for range of motion exercises or ways to assist the patient to walk. The dietician may be consulted for a list of foods allowed on a 2 Gm. Na diet. The pharmacist may provide information related to a particular medication, and other data may be obtained from the literature. It is necessary to make a specific plan by which to collect additional data. This includes identification of exactly what data is to be gathered, how, when, and from what source.

Sometimes the cause of the problem needs to be determined in order to better define the problem. In addition, knowledge of the cause of the problem could be influential in facilitating the management of the problem. For instance, referring to the example given in Chapter 6, The Problem List, the original problem statement defines the problem as "atrophy of adipose tissue of anterior upper thighs." In order to devise a plan for preventing further atrophy of tissue, the nurse needs to determine the cause of the atrophy. The available data base reveals that the patient is diabetic and that he gives himself daily injections of Regular Insulin. An analysis of the problem uncovers knowledge that atrophy of adipose tissue can result from failure to rotate injection sites and from injecting refrigerated insulin. The nurse cannot simply assume that the atrophy of tissue is caused by either factor alone or by both factors acting together. However, she can attempt to determine whether or not one or both factors (or neither) could be valid causes of the problem. The nurse can gather additional data from the patient pertaining to: 1) where he stores the vial of insulin presently in use, 2) whether or not he injects refrigerated (cold) insulin, and 3) the site(s) he uses for injection. In the "plan" section of the initial plan, the nurse would write specific directions as follows:

> *Plan:* Will talk c̄ patient this afternoon to determine cause of tissue atrophy. Will ask patient: 1) where he stores his insulin, 2) *if* refrigerated, whether or not he injects insulin taken from the refrigerator or at room temperature, and 3) to describe where (site) he injects insulin.

Since this nurse planned to execute this part of the plan herself, it was not necessary to identify who should collect the data. Had she planned to delegate this task, the nurse would have stated who would be responsible for obtaining the information.

Plans for dissemination of information

These plans may take many forms and involve a variety of individuals.

1. Information may have to be given to the patient concerning what he needs and wants to know about his illness, and what he is expected to do. For example, specific directions may pertain to medication, activities, or foods to be eaten or avoided.
2. Information has to be given to family members or other significant individuals explaining how they may assist the patient in managing his illness or what they must do to assume the responsibility for his care.
3. Pertinent data may need to be reported to the physician or other members of the health team.
4. Upon discharge from a hospital, information or instructions may have to be given to nursing personnel in other agencies such as a Public Health Department or Visiting Nurse Association. Depending on the anticipated length of hospitalization, this may or may not be included in the initial plan.

Plans for the dissemination of information must state precisely what information is to be imparted to whom, how, when, and by whom. When appropriate, the plan should include what is expected of the individual as a result of receiving the information. It is essential that the plans be as specific as possible. It is not sufficient to state that one is planning to talk with the patient about his illness; it is necessary to know exactly *what* the patient will be told. By indicating this on the chart, anyone dealing with the patient should be better able to reinforce what he has already been told, or at least not contradict the approach of other health personnel. This consistency among members of the health team helps the patient feel more secure about the individuals responsible for him and his care. Examples of plans for giving information are:

Plan: Beginning on 4-3-73, patient's nursing student will: 1) explain the purpose for coughing and deep breathing after surgery and 2) instruct patient in how to deep breathe and cough using abdominal muscles preparatory to what will be expected of him postoperatively.

Plan: Will talk c̄ patient's wife on 4-10-73 to review range of motion exercises she can perform for patient at home.

Treatment plans

The treatment plan is the statement of nursing care objectives pertinent to a given problem and the prescription of nursing orders designed to achieve these objectives. The plans may concern maintenance or restoration of the patient's usual patterns, alleviation of symptoms arising from the problem, and/or prevention of complications or additional problems.

Nursing Care Objectives. The *purposes* of nursing care objectives are:

1. To provide a means of evaluating nursing care
2. To serve as a channel of communication between patient, family, and members of the health team
3. To guide in making decisions pertaining to the management of problems
4. To provide focus for nursing care
5. To provide standards for measuring patient progress
6. To state behavior which will indicate that nursing objectives have been achieved.

A nursing care objective is defined as *an intent communicated by a statement describing a specific behavior (or patterns of behavior) which the nurse expects the patient to demonstrate as a result of nursing intervention.* However, in some instances, the behavior described may be that expected to be performed by the family or some other person significant to the patient. At other times, the behavior may be physiologic and thus concerned with the blood pressure, the decubitus ulcer, the bowels, and so on. Other definitions pertinent to writing nursing care objectives are:

1. Behavior—any visible activity displayed by a patient.
2. Terminal behavior—that behavior which the nurse expects the patient to demonstrate as a result of the nursing methods employed in his care.
3. Criterion—a standard or test by which the terminal behavior is evaluated.[5]

According to Mager, terminal behavior is best described by:

1. Identifying the exact *behavior* that will be accepted as evidence that the expected outcome was achieved.
2. Defining the important *conditions* under which the behavior is to occur.
3. Specifying the *criterion* of acceptable performance.[6]

Components of Behavioral Objectives. As stated above, a nursing care objective includes a statement of the *behavior* expected to be demonstrated, the *conditions* under which the behavior is expected to occur, and the *criterion* for determining acceptable performance. Each of these components will be discussed in detail along with an additional component, the *subject*.

1. When writing nursing care objectives, it is necessary to state the *subject* expected to demonstrate the specified behavior. This will usually be the patient, but could be a family member or other significant person. At other times, the nurse may expect certain physiologic behavior and in these instances objectives are written with the subject identified as the skin, the blood pressure, the weight, and so on.

2. *Behavior* results from a combination of influences and is usually a mixture of these four major types: 1) psychomotor, 2) affective, 3) cognitive, and 4) physiologic. *Psychomotor behavior* is that involving control of muscles. Examples include walking, feeding, writing, and talking. *Affective behavior* is that concerned with feelings and attitudes. For example, expression of fear or anger. *Cognitive behavior* involves the use of the intellectual processes such as remembering, understanding, and problem solving. Examples are listing pros and cons of a regimen and making a decision. *Physiologic activity* is behavior of the bodily processes, such as healing of broken skin, bowel elimination, sleep, and temperature control.

Only a verb can be used to express the expected behavior. Whenever possible, verbs stating specific overt behavior should be used. For example, verbs such as write, walk, talk, inject, and decrease are preferable to such terms as know, understand, be comfortable, and be better. There are times when the nurse must use vague terms because no others completely describe the behavior she expects the patient to demonstrate. In these instances, she must further define the behavior by stating how the subject will demonstrate that the objective has been achieved. For example, she may write "Patient will know _____ as evidenced by _____."

Since the nursing care objective describes expected behavior, it should be written in positive rather than negative terms. The behavior is stated in terms of what will be achieved, not what will be avoided.

A common mistake is stating "Patient will have _____." Anytime the words "will have" are used, someone other than the subject will be performing the behavior. This is incorrect, as the objective is intended to communicate the behavior of the subject. For example, stating "Patient will move his bowels daily before noon," is preferable to "Patient will have a bowel movement daily before noon."

3. In order to define the terminal behavior it is often necessary to state the *conditions* under which this behavior is expected to be demonstrated. Including the conditions in an objective helps to clarify exactly what is expected of the subject. Conditions may be either "givens" or "restrictions" which serve to structure the circumstances of the terminal behavior.

Givens	*Restrictions*
With assistance	Without assistance
Using a schedule	Within one hour
Using a walker	While in the hospital

For example, an objective stating, "Patient will walk the length of the hall q.i.d. without assistance," gives a picture of quite different behavior than an objective reading, "Using his walker, patient will walk the length of the hall q.i.d."

A condition is not necessary for every objective. It is used only to make the terminal behavior more explicit. The important thing to remember is that the condition structures the circumstances under which the behavior is to be performed and, thus, must be evident *at the time the behavior is performed*. For example, in the objective "Given instructions prior to discharge, the patient will test his urine for sugar and acetone q.d. at home and record the results," the condition is incorrectly stated as it does not describe the conditions under which the urine testing is to occur. However, in the objective, "Using the two-drop method, patient will test urine for sugar and acetone q.d. at home and record the results," the condition, "using the two-drop method," clarifies the actual performance of the behavior.

4. Describing the *criterion* of acceptable performance also aids in clarifying terminal behavior. This standard for comparison should specify at

least the minimum performance acceptable as evidence that the objective has been achieved. The criterion may be stated as a minimum number of times a behavior will be performed in a given length of time, a minimum number of responses, or a time limit. Examples include: each morning, one pound per week, and 40 feet, three times daily.

While each of the items for defining terminal behavior (the subject, behavior, condition, and criterion) helps make an objective more specific, it is not always necessary to include all of them. The subject and behavior must always be stated to know who is expected to do what. There are times when the condition and/or criterion may be omitted. However, some statement of criterion is necessary to evaluate *how well* the subject performed the expected behavior. Therefore, nursing care objectives should almost always contain three items: subject, behavior, and criterion. Conditions should state when necessary for clarification of the circumstances under which the terminal behavior is to be demonstrated. Examples of nursing care objectives followed by a breakdown of their component parts are:

1. Using a walker, the patient will walk at least 40 feet t.i.d.
   Subject—the patient
   Behavior—will walk
   Condition—using a walker
   Criterion—at least 40 feet t.i.d.
2. The patient will lose 10 pounds within 2 weeks.
   Subject—the patient
   Behavior—will lose pounds
   Condition—none
   Criterion—10 within 2 weeks.
3. Temperature will remain below 37.6° C.
   Subject—temperature
   Behavior—will remain below 37.6° C.
   Condition—none
   Criterion—none
4. Ankle edema will decrease as evidenced by measurement below 28 cm.
   Subject—ankle edema
   Behavior—will decrease
   Condition—none
   Criterion—as evidenced by measurement below 28 cm.
5. Using the two-drop method, the patient will test his urine for sugar and acetone q.i.d. and record the results.
   Subject—the patient
   Behavior—will test his urine for sugar and acetone and record the results.

Condition—using the two-drop method
Criterion—q.i.d.
6. The patient will sleep more comfortably between 2400 and 0600 hours as evidenced by no more than two episodes of shortness of breath each night.
   Subject—the patient
   Behavior—will sleep more comfortably between 2400 and 0600 hours
   Condition—none
   Criterion—as evidenced by no more than two episodes of shortness of breath each night.
7. The patient will discuss her labor experience with her nurse within 24 hours after delivery.
   Subject—the patient
   Behavior—will discuss her labor experience with her nurse
   Condition—none
   Criterion—within 24 hours after delivery.

Because nursing deals with meeting immediate needs, the nursing care objectives advocated (such as those written above) tend to illustrate more short-term or immediate aims. In addition, we are more able to evaluate progress (or lack of it) when we have short-term objectives. The evaluation of achievement of long-term objectives requires an extended time period and nurses do not usually see patients over a long period of time. This is especially true in a referral hospital where most of the patients are from out of town.

There are times, however, when our intent can only be made known through the statement of a long-term objective. When this is the case, the objective (like any other objective) needs to include a description of the terminal behavior the patient is to demonstrate. Then, to allow for evaluation of progress, the terminal behavior may need to be broken down into component tasks, each of which must be mastered as a prerequisite to demonstrating the terminal behavior. Another way is to write an objective for each of a series of steps leading to the terminal behavior. In other words, an objective would have to be written to describe the expected outcome of each step. Thus, some behavior is expected to be demonstrated for each of the steps leading to the terminal behavior.

In summary, the primary purpose for stating nursing care objectives in patient behavioral terms is to provide a means of evaluating patient progress and the effect of nursing care on the patient. Nursing care is evaluated in terms of whether or not it achieved what it set out to do—that is, whether we "get to where we are going" in managing or solving the patient's nursing problems or whether we do not. Thus, we advocate the planning of short-term nursing care objectives which are intended to meet immediate needs rather than long-term objectives which usually cannot begin to be evaluated during an average hospital stay. In addition to providing a means of evaluation, however, nursing care objectives serve several other useful functions:

1. Nursing care objectives are a means of communicating to the patient and the family, to other members of the nursing staff as well as to other members of the health team, exactly what is to be achieved in order to manage or solve a particular nursing problem.

Objectives may originate with either the patient and/or family or with the nurse. Regardless of how they originate, objectives require the active (whenever possible) participation of both the patient (and family) and the nurse to be achieved. Objectives are discussed with the patient periodically (the frequency depending upon the problem) and may be modified at any time, again with both the patient and the nurse participating. We have found that when the patient knows what is expected of him and is given a chance to participate in planning his nursing care, we seem to have fewer problems or complications during his hospital stay as well as a patient who has, or at least expresses, more positive feelings related to the nursing care he receives.

Because they state our intent or aim, nursing care objectives communicate what we are trying to do in order to manage a particular problem to other members of the nursing staff as well as to other members of the health team. Thus, objectives may serve to provide for some degree of continuity and consistency between the various members of the health team dealing with the patient and his problems.

2. The statement of a nursing care objective may serve as a useful guide in making a decision as to what methods need to be ordered to manage or solve the problem.

3. The stated objectives help the nursing staff and/or nursing students to focus the nursing care they give.

4. Closely related to evaluation itself, behaviorally stated nursing care objectives provide the criteria by which progress is determined. Prior knowledge of the criteria by which progress is determined tells us what to look for and, thus, can be of assistance in identifying pertinent information to record in progress notes. This knowledge can also serve as a guide to help us see the need for modification of a part or of the entire plan.

5. Nursing care objectives stating the expected terminal behavior enable us to identify when we have arrived at our destination. Being able to see that we have accomplished what we set out to do and see the effects of our efforts, allows for a feeling of success or completion which may otherwise never be felt. Nurses are constantly faced with feelings of guilt and/or inadequacy because they cannot "get everything done." Nursing care objectives won't necessarily get everything done, but they do break "everything" down into specific goals toward which she can usually achieve some progress. Nurses who have written nursing care objectives for their patients and then worked with these patients to meet the ob-

jectives feel that they obtain rewards which they do not otherwise receive. The rewards are mainly psychologic in nature, but they enable nurses to feel that something has been accomplished through their efforts and this, in turn, contributes to the feeling of having done a "good job"—a feeling which we all need.

Nursing Orders. A nursing order is defined as *the prescription of specific methods or directions by which nursing care objectives are to be achieved and which assist in the management and/or solution of patients' nursing problems.* They are prescribed by nurses, for nurses, and refer to patients' nursing care, not medical care.

Nursing orders are numbered to correspond with the nursing care objective for which they are designed, and thus are also keyed to the particular problem on the problem list. The nurse must decide whether one or several orders are needed to assist the patient with a specific problem. Other factors to be considered when selecting nursing methods are the safety and comfort of the patient, available staff and staff time, available equipment, cost of equipment, the organization of the particular unit, and, whenever safely allowed, the patient's preferences.

It is essential that nursing orders be written in such a way that any member of the health team reading them would know exactly what to do, how to do it, and when it should be done. For example, a nursing order stating "turn and position" is inadequate for management of the problem "reddened skin over sacrum." It is important to know the exact plan for positioning. Therefore, the nurse must indicate where the patient should be turned (i.e., to his right side, left side, back, or abdomen), when he should be turned, exactly how he should be positioned, and what should be used to keep him in the position indicated. It is often advisable to post a turning and positioning chart over the patient's bed stating how he should be positioned at what times.

Successful communication through written nursing orders is not an easy task. Cowan and McPherson state:

If you've never written any directions, you may think it's easier and more fun to tell someone else how to dig a ditch or scrub a floor than it is to do the digging or scrubbing yourself. But giving directions is not easy unless you know what you are doing. You have to understand two things: how to do whatever it is that you are telling someone else to do, and how to get that knowledge down on paper clearly enough so that your reader can follow your directions.[7]

There are many times when, in order to individualize a patient's care or determine the exact character and degree of assistance needed, the nurse must carry out the plan of care herself before she is able to communicate specific directions to others.

The nursing order must state the *behavior* to be performed by the reader or designated individual. Verbs stating specific overt actions should be used. For example: walk, tell, give, apply, record, and rub. Vague words such as reassure, support, and encourage should not be used since they are open to many interpretations. If such terms cannot be avoided the writer must specify exactly how the reader is to perform the behavior. The word "offer" should not be used unless the nurse wishes the patient to choose one of several alternatives.

The *recipient* of the action must also be included in the nursing order. This is usually the patient, but could be a family member or other significant person. When the recipient is clearly understood to be the patient, it is not necessary to state this in each order. Also, there are times when a particular part of the patient is to receive the nursing measure. For example, in the nursing order "Apply A and D ointment to lips q.i.d. at 1000, 1400, 1800, and 2200," the "lips" are the recipients.

The *object* of the nursing order describes *what* is to be given, applied, told, and so on. For example, in the order, "Give patient warm milk q.d. h.s.," the object is "warm milk." Also included is *how* the behavior is to be performed, such as "according to fluid plan at bedside."

The *frequency* and specific *time* at which the order is to be carried out must also be stated. This may be expressed as a clock hour (0900), in relation to other activity (after breakfast), or by statements such as "on even hours," or "on odd hours while awake."

Depending on the particular nursing order, there are occasions when the recipient or object may be omitted. However, the behavior and time should always be stated. Examples of nursing orders followed by a breakdown of their component parts are:

1. Give hot coffee q.d. at 0700.
   Behavior—give
   Recipient—understood to be the patient
   Object—hot coffee
   Time—q.d. at 0700
2. Show Mrs. Green (patient's daughter) procedure for decubitus care on 7-1-73 during afternoon visiting hours.
   Behavior—show
   Recipient—Mrs. Green
   Object—procedure for decubitus care
   Time—on 7-1-73 during afternoon visiting hours
3. Give all pills and capsules with applesauce.
   Behavior—give
   Recipient—understood to be the patient
   Object—pills and capsules with applesauce
   Time—understood to be whenever pills and capsules are given
4. Elevate head of bed 90° when giving fluids, medications, and meals.

Behavior—elevate 90°
Recipient—head of bed
Object—none
Time—when giving fluids, medications, and meals
5. Turn patient q2h (even) and position according to turning plan at bedside.
Behavior—turn and position
Recipient—patient
Object—according to turning plan
Time—q2h
6. Rub back with lotion at 2200.
Behavior—rub
Recipient—back
Object—with lotion
Time—at 2200.
7. Hold patient's hand and walk with him from his bed to the nursing station and back to bed q.d. at 1000, 1400, and 1900.
Behavior—hold hand and walk
Recipient—patient (could be omitted)
Object—from his bed to the nursing station and back to bed
Time—q.d. at 1000, 1400, and 1900.
8. Record patient's pulse and respiratory rates before and after walking.
Behavior—record
Recipient—pulse and respiratory rates
Object—none
Time—before and after walking.
9. Apply Calamine Lotion to rash on back q.i.d. at 1000, 1400, 1800, and 2200.
Behavior—apply
Recipient—rash on back
Object—Calamine Lotion
Time—q.i.d. at 1000, 1400, 1800, and 2200.

SUMMARY

Each nursing problem should have its own plan identified by the same number and title use on the problem list. The discussion of the initial plan for each problem should take into consideration the data found in the patient's Nursing History pertaining to his usual life style, preferences, and coping patterns, as well as information obtained by other members of the health team, including the medical diagnosis, medical plan of care, laboratory results, and so on. The plan is the result of thorough analysis of each problem and its interrelationship with others. The format to be followed for recording the initial plan is:

Problem number and title

Subjective data: information relative to the given problem from the patient's point of view.

Objective data: facts (quantitative when possible) relative to the stated problem derived from the nurse's observations.

Assessment: summarization of the nurse's thoughts regarding the problem.

Plan: the specific design, method, or scheme of action by which the given problem is to be managed. It may consist of:

1. Plans for the collection of additional data to better define the problem or facilitate its management. This includes identification of specific data to be gathered, how, when, and by whom.
2. Plans for the dissemination of information pertinent to management of the problem. This includes directions stating what information is to be given, how, when, and by whom. When appropriate, indicate what is expected of the patient (or others) as a result of having been given particular information.
3. Plans for nursing treatment of the problem. This involves delineation of nursing care objectives and prescription of nursing orders designed to meet them.

DIRECTIONS FOR WRITING THE INITIAL PLAN

1. Title the plan "Initial Plan."
2. Record the date on which the initial plan is written.
3. Place the initial plan in the patient's chart following the problem list.
4. Number and title each plan to correspond with the number and title of the problem on the problem list to which it pertains. A plan must be related to a problem identified on the problem list.
5. Record the following elements for each problem:
   a. A discussion of each problem including the subjective and objective data which contributed to the nurse's identification of the problem
   b. An assessment of each problem reflecting the nurse's thoughts about the problem
   c. A plan.
6. Record the above elements of the initial plan under the four headings of:
   a. Subjective data
   b. Objective data
   c. Assessment
   d. Plan.
7. Include all of the above headings in each plan even if it is necessary to state "none" or "nothing at this time" beside it.
8. State all pertinent data which contributed to the identification of the problem (derived from Nursing History, family or significant others, and

100

other members of the health team) under the appropriate heading of subjective or objective data.

9. Identify factors which may enhance or inhibit the management or solution of the problem and discuss these factors under the assessment section of each plan.

10. State the plan for the management or solution of each problem indicating whether the plan is intended to collect additional data, to give information to others, or to treat the existing problem.

11. Make certain that each plan is consistent with the medical plan of care.

12. Base each plan on scientific knowledge, utilizing research whenever possible.

13. Write each plan for the present; i.e., write only plans that deal with immediate needs or problems. Do not write postoperative plans until the patient is in that stage. Do not write plans for future needs or problems unless the plan includes a sequence of steps; then, all steps may be written at one time.

14. State the following for each plan to collect additional data:
   a. Exactly what data is to be collected
   b. How
   c. When
   d. By whom.

15. Identify the following for each plan to disseminate information:
   a. Exactly what information is to be given to whom
   b. How
   c. When
   d. By whom
   e. When appropriate, what is expected of the individual to whom the information will be given as a result of having received it.

16. State the nursing care objective for each treatment plan when some behavior is expected to be demonstrated by the patient as a result of nursing intervention.

17. Number each objective to correspond with the number of the problem for which it is intended; such as Objective #3 for Problem #3. If more than one objective is written for one problem, record them as Objective #3a, Objective #3b. Objective #3c, and so on.

18. Include the following components in each nursing care objective when appropriate.
   a. The subject who is to perform the expected behavior
   b. The terminal behavior (specific action verb)
   c. The conditions under which behavior will occur
   d. The criterion for determining acceptable performance.

Note: All objectives will not contain a condition and/or criterion; however, the terminal expected outcome can be made more specific when all four components are included in each objective.

19. Write each nursing care objective in terms of the expected behavior to be performed by the subject.

20. Write each nursing care objective in positive behavioral terms rather than in negative terms.

21. Write the nursing orders by which to achieve each nursing care objective.

22. Number each nursing order to correspond with the number of each objective (and in turn for each problem) for which it is written; such as Order #3 for Objective #3 or Order #3a for Objective #3a. If more than one order is written for one objective, record them as Order #3-1 or Order #3a-1.

23. Include the following components in each nursing order:
   a. The activity to be performed (specific action verb)
   b. The subject who is to receive the action (the recipient). It is not necessary to state the recipient when it is clearly understood to be the patient.
   c. The object or *what* is to be given, recorded, applied, and so on, and *how* the activity is to be performed unless there are standards already devised for the performance of the activity.
   d. The time or times the activity is to be performed.

24. Sign the initial plan.

REFERENCES

1. Mager, Robert F.: *Preparing Instructional Objectives*. Fearon Publishers, Inc., Palo Alto, 1962, p. vii.
2. Weed, Lawrence L.: "Medical records, patient care, and medical education." *Irish Journal of Medical Science* 6:272, 1964.
3. Weed, Lawrence L.: *Medical Records, Medical Education and Patient Care*. The Press of Case Western Reserve University, Cleveland, Year Book Medical Publishers, Inc., Chicago, 1969, p. 50.
4. Ibid., p. 43.
5. Mager, op. cit., p. 2.
6. Ibid., p. 12.
7. Cowan, Gregory, and McPherson, Elisabeth: *Plain English Please*. Random House, New York, 1966, p. 41.

8

PROGRESS NOTES

The information necessary for evaluating progress achieved in the management of nursing problems is recorded in the progress notes, the fourth phase of the problem-oriented system. Evaluation of nursing care can be discussed only in terms of defined goals, standards, and specifications. Thus, progress notes may be defined as *a written record describing developments in a predetermined plan of nursing care.*

Traditionally, nursing notes have consisted of a series of insufficiently informative statements about what was done for the patient or comments expressing value judgments without data to support the opinions of the nurse. For example, "dressing changed," "walked in hall," "up in chair," "seems better," "ate well," and "slept well." Nursing care cannot be evaluated on the basis of such information. Notes should include answers to such questions as: What was the appearance of the wound? How far did the patient walk? Did he experience any difficulties? How long did the patient sit in a chair? Did he require any assistance? What observations indicated that the patient was better? Better than what? What exactly did the patient eat? How did he feel after eating? How long did he sleep before awakening? What was his opinion concerning the quality of this sleep? In addition, it is usually incorrect to state medications given and vital signs in the nursing notes since this information is recorded on special sheets elsewhere in the patient's chart. However, there are times when such notations may be significant. For example. the nurse may record a blood pressure or temperature reading which is unusual for the particular patient and which she thinks requires further observation. It is unnecessary and repetitive to include such information in nursing notes just for the sake of having something to write at the end of the shift.

Progress notes written according to the guidelines given in this text provide useful data for evaluating progress and planning the management of patients' nursing problems. They will also supply records which can be used for the development of criteria to determine effective patient care, to better predict outcomes of the utilization of particular methods of nursing care, and to teach students of nursing.

Weed states that progress notes are the most crucial part of the patient's record because "they are the mechanism of follow-up on each problem."[1] They reveal the current status of the problem and the progress (or lack of it) made toward its solution. Systematically written progress notes provide constant feedback of information which assists the nurse to better define the problem and, in light of up-to-date evidence, alter the plan of management in a manner that enhances the possibility of solving the problem. These notes also contain all additional data acquired and any resulting modification of plans. If the data yield a new problem, this should be added to the problem list and an adequate definition recorded in a progress note. Each note should relate directly to the problem list by stating the number and title of the problem to which it pertains.

Information included in the notes may be obtained from: 1) the nurse's own observations, 2) statements made by the patient and/or family, 3) reports made by other members of the health team, 4) data obtained from check lists, flow sheets, laboratory reports, diagnositc and treatment procedures, and X-rays, and 5) research reports and other scientific literature. A review of the complete problem list, all plans, and previous progress notes relevant to the given problem should be made before writing a note or modifying plans for the management of a problem. A daily review of each active problem helps to ensure that ". . . a maximum effort is being exerted to resolve it, as opposed to an aimless collection of further information of questionable utility."[2] Weed also states:

Frequently, earlier evidence . . . is neither supported nor refuted; it is never interpreted or even appreciated. It is ignored. Often these data were obtained at great discomfort and expense to the patient and, if studied, may provide the evidence needed to solve the patient's current problems.[3]

This follow-up procedure is the most difficult part of the process to implement. Evaluation is never easy and the progress notes record constant evaluation of the nurse's thought process, the plans she makes using her cognitive skills, and the results of implementing these plans. In addition, this evaluation is placed in the patient's chart for all to see. However, developing the skills required to write useful progress notes and effectively utilize them is essential for proper management of nursing care problems.

KINDS OF PROGRESS NOTES

Progress notes are divided into two categories: 1) narrative notes, and 2) flow sheets. In the remainder of this text, the term "progress note" refers

104

to the narrative variety. While the flow sheet is a type of progress note, it will always be specifically referred to as a flow sheet.

NARRATIVE PROGRESS NOTE

The progress notes are recorded in chronological order following the formulation of the initial plan. They are dated and titled "Nursing Progress Note." (The title may be needed only when all members of the health team record their progress notes in the same section of the patient's chart.) These notes are used to record the patient's response to the plans for the management of each problem. They also describe data leading to the identification of new problems, assessments of progress made in light of the patient's response to the plan, and a statement of future plans for the management of the problem. Thus, any addition, deletion, or modification in the plan of care is included in the progress notes.

Each note consists of four major sections identical to those of the initial plan:

1. Subjective data
2. Objective data
3. Assessment
4. Plan.

These will be discussed in the section titled "Components of Nursing Progress Notes."

FLOW SHEET

The flow sheet is a graphic representation of significant data pertinent to the patient's problems as identified on the problem list. There are times when a narrative progress note is not an adequate method of recording data. This is especially true as we attempt to relate multiple variables or determine existing relationships in available data.[4] Usually the flow sheet is used in conjunction with narrative progress notes; however, there are times when the flow sheet may be the only progress note written. This occurs primarily in crisis situations where the status of the problem is rapidly changing.

The nurse must decide: 1) which problems should have a flow sheet, 2) which parameters to include, and 3) the frequency with which the variables should be followed. It is essential to provide an appropriate space for entering the data (and time, when necessary) on the flow sheet. According to Weed: "The time required initially in setting up a proper flow sheet is small compared to that wasted unraveling and reassembling disorganized and misplaced data."[5]

105

Flow sheets are most frequently used to record repetitive data such as vital signs, daily weights, fluid intake and output, and medications. They may describe wound drainage and healing, size of decubitus ulcers, degree of ankle edema, or occurrence of urinary or fecal incontinence. They may indicate whether the patient feeds and dresses himself or requires nursing assistance, and whether he or the nurse administers his insulin injections. Flow sheets are especially useful when time relationships may be significant. For example, one may observe at a glance that the days when a patient was extremely hypotensive coincided with those days when large amounts of fluid were lost through diarrhea and vomiting, that the times the patient complained of a headache occurred on those days when the patient's husband visited, or that asthma attacks took place on those days the patient was told by his physician that he was doing better and would be able to go home soon. Depending upon the problem, it is possible to combine the idea of the check list and that of the flow sheet. In this manner, the nurse can see at a glance what has been done for the problem and the progress made as a result. This is particularly useful when, for example, the nurse is trying different methods of mouth care or decubitus ulcer care and wants a picture of the results yielded by the various methods.

WRITING NURSING PROGRESS NOTES

The question is often asked "How frequently should a progress note be written?" Nurses have traditionally written notes at the end of each shift. However, a progress note is not the same thing as the traditional shift report or shift nursing note. There is no set rule stating how often a progress note should be written. Depending upon the circumstances, it may be recorded every hour, several times during a shift, once a day, or once a week. Factors affecting the frequency include: 1) the data being collected, 2) the criterion for frequency stated in the nursing care objective, 3) the rate of change in a patient's condition, 4) any occurrences which give rise to new data, and 5) the number of occasions on which a patient volunteers new information. These latter two situations occur frequently during a patient's hospitalization. The patient's daily response to routine tests and procedures affords much valuable information to an attentive nurse. When the nurse strives to know her patient, and the patient feels that a particular nurse is *his* nurse, hardly a day passes without some new information being discovered.

COMPONENTS OF NURSING PROGRESS NOTES

The parts of the nursing progress note include the title, time, problem number and title, subjective data, objective data, assessment, future plans, and the nurse's signature.

Date and Time. The nurse should record the date and time the progress note is written. For example: 3-16-73 (1015). Since notes are recorded as

106

needed, and not merely at the end of a shift, the time indicates when the data was obtained as well as when the note was written. Statement of the date and time aids in determining the sequence and interrelationships of noted developments. Also, the date of modification, resolution, or addition of a problem on the problem list should correspond with the date of the progress note containing the information upon which this decision was based.

Title "Nursing Progress Note." This title is optional. When the progress notes of all members of the health team are kept together in one section of the patient's chart, it is necessary to have the note designated as a *nursing* progress note. However, in institutions where a separate section of the patient's chart is used for nursing notes it is unnecessary to include this title each time a note is written.

Problem Number and Title. This is the notation of the problem number and title, as stated on the problem list, to which the progress note pertains. For example: Problem #3—Pain. If one progress note is concerned with data relevant to several problems, each problem should be listed and discussed separately.

Subjective Data. This section of the progress note consists of information relative to the problem from the patient's point of view. Subjective data is that which the patient reports. This may include his opinion of what is being done for him, what else he thinks should be done, how he reports he is feeling, and any thoughts he has about the problem. Examples include:

1. Feels more "nervous" (jittery, irritable) today.
2. "Can't eat this food without salt."
3. Requests laxative.
4. "Can't stand much more of this pain."

Objective Data. This is the factual information resulting from the nurse's observations pertinent to the given problem. Whenever possible, objective data should reflect quantitative observations or measurements. What is being done for the problem (medically and/or nursing) may be included, especially if this is a new occurrence or plan, or when this knowledge enhances understanding of the patient's response. Examples are:

1. Present size of a decubitus ulcer.
2. Patient's present weight; notation of increase or decrease and period of time in which this occurred.
3. Results of a kidney biopsy.
4. Frequency with which pain medication is given.

Assessment. This section of the progress note is a summarization of the nurse's thoughts pertaining to a given problem. It may consist of:

1. Analysis of the nature of the problem in the light of new data.
2. Identification of factors enhancing or inhibiting progress in managing the problem.
3. Thoughts about the patient's ability to participate or cooperate in his care, including assessment of his understanding of instructions and/or explanations.
4. Statement of the present status of the problem and the effect of nursing intervention to date.
5. Reasons for decision to continue, modify, or delete the present plan of management.

Assessment demonstrates the cognitive processes underlying the course of action taken by the nurse as she attempts to find the most effective, safe, and comfortable (for the patient) methods to manage patients' nursing problems.

Plan. This is the statement of plans for management of the problem in view of the most up-to-date information available to the nurse. In order to be effective, the plan of nursing care must be revised according to the patient's progress and as new information becomes available. Any changes or additions to the former plan are stated in this section of the progress note. The relationship between all parts of the progress note should be obvious. The reader should be able to see the data pertinent to the problem, the nurse's thought process, and the resulting plan. Plans delineated for each problem are categorized as:

1. Plans for collection of additional data to better define the problem or facilitate its management,
2. Plans for dissemination of information pertinent to management of the problem, and/or
3. Plans for the nursing "treatment" or management of the given problem.

Discussion of these categories appeared in Chapter 7, "The Initial Plan" to which the reader should refer for a review of this information.

Signature and Title. This is simply the signing of the note by the person writing it and his or her title. For example: C. Creen, R.N. Since the patient's chart may be used as legal evidence, each person writing in it should be able to account for the information he records.

SUMMARY

Progress notes recorded in the manner described supply specific data pertinent to the problem under consideration, plans for management of the problem, and the results of implementing these plans. This information is easily available to all members of the health team for review and coordination of their various efforts for managing the patient's problems. Progress notes provide the data necessary for evaluation of the nurse's thought process and actual nursing care procedures. The organization of problem-oriented progress notes reminds the writer ". . . to think systematically about a patient and provides evidence of whether he has actually done so."[6] Weed states that "The nature and extent of any incompleteness is immediately discernible in records containing an honest list of problems and accurately titled progress notes."[7] Only through effective evaluation and modification can nursing care be improved and nursing goals achieved.

DIRECTIONS FOR WRITING NURSING PROGRESS NOTES

1. Title each note "Nursing Progress Note."
2. Record the date and time at which the note is written.
3. Record each note in chronological order.
4. Write all information in a problem-oriented manner.
5. Number and subtitle all notes with the number and title of the problem on the problem list to which it pertains.
6. Include all of these elements in each note: Subjective Data, Objective Data, Assessment, and Plan.
7. State all pertinent data under the appropriate headings of subjective or objective data.
8. State data in terms of the patient's response to what was done, rather than in terms of what the nurse has done. Include the latter only when it contributes to a better understanding of the patient's response.
9. Include any of these in the assessment section:
   A. Analysis of nature of problem in view of newly obtained data.
   B. Identification of factors enhancing or inhibiting progress.
   C. Statement of the present status of the problem and the effect of nursing intervention to date.
   D. Evaluation of the patient's ability to participate or cooperate in his care, including an assessment of his understanding of instructions given.
   E. Reasons for decision to continue, modify, or delete the present plan of management.
10. State plans for management of each problem, indicating whether the present plan is to be continued, deleted, or modified (follow directions 10 through 23 given in Chapter 7).
11. Number and add each new problem to problem list with date of progress note containing data defining the problem.
12. Whenever a problem title is modified, write date in appropriate column on problem list to correspond to date of progress note containing information clarifying the problem.
13. Whenever a problem is resolved, write date of resolution in appropriate column on problem list to correspond to date of progress note containing data upon which this decision was based.

109

14. When additional data lead to identification of a new problem, follow directions 5 through 24 given in Chapter 7.

15. Sign each progress note using name and title.

EXAMPLES OF NURSING PROGRESS NOTES

5-30-73 (1000) Nursing Progress Note
Problem #3—Fluid Restriction
  Subjective data: Fluid plan helps as now knows when can have more fluid.
  Objective data: Is drinking amount of fluid at times specified on fluid plan. Total intake on 5-29-73 was 690 cc.
  Assessment: Fluid plan achieving goal of restricting fluid intake to 700 cc.
  Plan: Continue present plan.

C. Green, R.N.

2-26-73 (1400) Nursing Progress Note
Problem #2—Obesity
  Subjective data: States not as upset about diet as found that "I can eat a lot of things but in smaller portions."
  Objective data: Talked with dietician; given list of foods and portions allowed on 1500 calorie diet and exchange list.
  Assessment: Losing weight on diet; weight decreased from 114.2 kg. on admission to 111.8 kg. today. Believe that patient will work at staying on diet if she understands it.
  Plan:
    1. Review exchange list with patient on 2-27-73.
    2. Ask patient to make 2 sample menus for each meal (breakfast, lunch, dinner) using exchange list by 3-1-73.

E. Brown, R.N.

2-1-73 (1400) Nursing Progress Note
Problem #7—Edema
  Subjective data: Swelling in legs and feet is "almost gone." "They don't hurt so much now."
  Objective data: Measurements (at marks) have decreased as follows: left ankle 24 cm. to 21 cm., left knee 38 cm. to 33 cm., right ankle 25 cm. to 22 cm., right knee 40 cm. to 35 cm. Weight loss of another 0.5 kg. since yesterday.
  Assessment: With adherence to fluid plan, edema and weight are decreasing. No evidence of sacral edema. As edema appears to be gone, or at least markedly decreased, it seems time to begin getting patient out of bed and walking.

110

Plan:
1. Continue present plan.
2. Talk with physician about possibility of getting patient out of bed and walking. Need new activity order.

D. Loring, R.N.

3-28-73 (0830) Nursing Progress Note
Problem #1—Insulin administration

Subjective data: Awakened two-three times during night thinking about giving shot. "I'm really scared." After giving injection stated, "It wasn't so bad. There's nothing to that. I'll be able to do it again tomorrow because it didn't hurt at all."

Objective data: Prior to giving injection, patient had tears in her eyes; after giving injection, she was smiling.

Assessment: Able to draw up accurate dosage of insulin and inject it using proper technique. Knows about site rotation and how to locate correct injection sites. I believe patient will be able to adjust to giving self injections but still needs to acknowledge and express her feelings related to having to depend on insulin and giving self injections daily.

Plan:
1. Talk with patient at 1400 today about feelings related to having to give self injections.
2. Leave note in Kardex to have patient give own insulin on 3-29-73.
3. Record patient's reaction prior to and after giving injection.

S. White, R.N.

2-2-73 (1100) Nursing Progress Note
Problem #4—Weakness

Subjective data: Doesn't feel as weak. Believes that weakness will completely go away now that allowed out of bed.

Objective data: Ambulated in room by grabbing onto wall, curtains, bed, chair, etc., with one hand while holding onto me with other. No signs of physical distress.

Assessment: Still so weak that ambulation without more assistance (such as a walker or two people to walk her) seems unsafe at this time.

Plan:
1. Delete previous order #1 for ambulation.
2. Order walker from Physical Therapy.
3. Sit patient in chair t.i.d. for meals at 0800, 1200, and 1700. Return to bed after meals.
4. Walk patient to Nursing Station and back to bed with two people (one supporting each side) b.i.d. (1000 and 1400).

D. Loring, R.N.

Examples of progress notes concerned with new information related to problems already identified on the problem list:

10-23-73 (1015) Nursing Progress Note
Problem #3—Depression
Additional Information
> *Subjective data:* Wishes to die; can't take "this weakness" any longer. "I don't know what I want. I can't make a decision anymore."
>
> *Objective data:* Tears in eyes; lying rigid with arms at sides with fists clenched.
>
> *Assessment:* First mention of dying. May be fear of dying or realization that hers is a chronic condition and she may never feel "well" again. May be necessary to limit or eliminate decision making for a time, but will collect more information before making plans to do this.
>
> *Plan:* Will talk with patient this afternoon to obtain more information. Will begin by sitting down, extending my hand for her to hold and stating that I've been thinking about her comment about wishing to die. If patient says nothing, 1) ask her about this comment and 2) ask which decisions in particular (if any) she feels unable to make.
>
> E. Brown, R.N.

6-2-73 (1300) Nursing Progress Note
Problem #3—Ascites
Additional Data: Liver biopsy scheduled for 6-4-73.
> *Subjective data:* "Afraid." Has never had a biopsy of any kind but friend told all about how "awful" they are.
>
> *Objective data:* Crying
>
> *Assessment:* Too upset to listen to explanations at this time. Since listened to a friend, may help later to hear about experience from Mrs. Lewis who tolerated procedure well and said it was not as bad as she thought it would be.
>
> *Plan:*
> 1. Talk with patient about her fears related to liver biopsy at 1600 today.
> 2. On 6-3-73 explain procedure for liver biopsy, including what she may expect and what will be expected of her.
> 3. Arrange for Mrs. Lewis (patient) to talk with patient on 6-3-73 about her experience with liver biopsy.
>
> C. Loring, R.N.

6-4-73 (1600) Nursing Progress Note
Problem #3—Fluid restriction
Additional Data: Fluid restriction changed to 1500 cc/day.
> *Subjective data:* Is "glad" about change.
>
> *Objective data:* Has lost desired weight; physician believes patient is possibly dehydrated.
>
> *Assessment:* Foresee no problem as long as patient and family have fluid plan to follow.
>
> *Plan:* Modify Objective #3 to: Patient will drink 1500 cc. fluid/day.

Orders:
1. Call dietary about increasing fluid on trays from 60 cc. to 120 cc. each meal.
2. Refer to fluid plan at bedside for amount of fluid and times she is to receive it.

D. Jones, R.N.

An example of a progress note for recording additional data leading to the identification of a new problem:

7-1-73 (1530) Nursing Progress Note
New Problem #5—Menstruation
   Subjective data: Not time for regular period; periods have been irregular for past 4 months "because of the menopause." No cramping or other discomfort.
   Objective data: Given peri-pads.
   Assessment: Since patient is on Heparin, the chance of hemmorrhage exists.
   Plan: Add New Problem #5—Menstruation, to problem list.
      1. Give patient paper and pencil and ask that she keep a record of the number of peri-pads used daily.
      2. Provide container in which patient may save peri-pads for the nurse's observation.
      3. Observe and note on above record whether pad is saturated or has moderate or scant amount of blood.

M. Smith, R.N.

The new information may be unrelated to a problem already identified on the problem list and may not yield identification of a new problem. However, the nurse may decide that it is necessary to collect additional information to make a decision about whether or not a problem exists and/or precisely what the problem is. An example of such a progress note is:

7-9-73 (0500) Nursing Progress Note
Additional Data
   Subjective data: Feels "tense and worried." "I don't know what is bothering me."
   Objective data: Awake at each hourly check during night; looked tearful 2 times.
   Assessment: Need more information. Believe that if patient knew I had time to sit and listen to her that she would talk.
   Plan:
      1. Tell patient this morning that I will be in at 1500 this afternoon and will have time to talk with her.
      2. Set aside 45 minutes and plan with staff not to be interrupted.

3. Sit by patient and ask if she has been able to identify what was upsetting her last night.
4. May refer to tearing.

E. Jones, R.N.

If the additional data suggests a one-time course of action or even a series of actions, but not a problem to be worked with over a period of time, it can be dealt with in the progress notes without being entered on the problem list. For example:

9-26-73 (1400) Nursing Progress Note
Additional Data
  Subjective data: Requests to see chaplain; is used to own pastor visiting when hospitalized in home town.
  Objective data: None.
  Assessment: Seems to be no problem other than being important to patient to see chaplain.
  Plan:
    1. Notify chaplain's office of patient's request to see him.
    2. Ask patient 9-27-73 if she has seen chaplain.
    3. If patient has not seen chaplain by 9-28-73 follow-up on request in order to give explanation to patient as to why chaplain has not been to see her.

D. Loring, R.N.

The following example illustrates how the plan of care is modified through the progress notes.

6-14-73 (0900) Nursing Progress Note
Problem #4—Mouth Sores
  Subjective data: Tongue and inside of mouth still sore. "Hurts so bad I can hardly eat."
  Objective data: Has been receiving mouth care with hydrogen peroxide (1 part hydrogen peroxide to 1 part water) and Cepacol mouthwash at least q.i.d. New sore noted on left lateral part of tongue appearing as an indentation measuring about ⅛ in. by ⅛ in. Otherwise mouth looks as described on 6-13-73.
  Assessment: Present plan of mouth care is not effective in healing the sores or in contributing to the patient's comfort. Present solution of hydrogen peroxide may be too strong considering the condition of the mucous membranes of the mouth. Also, in view of the soreness, patient seems to need a local anesthetic which may at least help her to be able to eat.
  Plan:
    1. Continue use of hydrogen peroxide, but in a weaker concentration. Modify order #1 to: Rinse mouth with hydrogen peroxide solu-

tion (1 part hydrogen peroxide to 3 parts water) followed by Cepacol mouthwash.

2. Request order for Viscous Xylocaine.

B. Woods, R.N.

REFERENCES

1. Weed, Lawrence L.: *Medical Records, Medical Education, and Patient Care.* The Press of Case Western Reserve University, Cleveland, Year Book Medical Publishers, Inc., Chicago, 1969, p. 49.
2. Ibid., p. 46.
3. Ibid., p. 53.
4. Weed, Lawrence L.: "Medical records that guide and teach." *The New England Journal of Medicine* 278:599, 1968.
5. Ibid., p. 599.
6. Weed, Lawrence L.: *Medical Records, Medical Education, and Patient Care.* The Press of Case Western Reserve University, Cleveland, Year Book Medical Publishers, Inc., Chicago, 1969, p. 53.
7. Ibid., p. 29.

9

THE DISCHARGE NOTE

This final phase of the problem-oriented system is a summary of the patient's nursing problems and recommendations for their future management. The nursing discharge note is written when the patient is discharged from the hospital, when he is transferred to another unit within the same hospital or to another institution or health facility. In the latter instance, it may be referred to as a transfer note. However, in the remainder of this text, the term discharge note will be used to include the transfer note. A separate section discusses the type of summary written when a patient expires.

In all instances, it is best if the note is written at the time of the occurrence; if circumstances prohibit this, it should be written within 24 hours. The discharge note should be problem-oriented and may be written using the same format as progress notes. It reviews all of the patient's nursing problems and includes a notation of those which were resolved and those which are active at the time of discharge. This requires that the nurse review the patient's chart and select relevant data from the Nursing History and progress notes. Since the emphasis is on active nursing problems, the discharge note should include that data base which defines a problem and indicates a need for nursing intervention, as well as information necessary for the future analysis or management of the problem.[1]

FUNCTIONS OF THE NURSING DISCHARGE NOTE

1. The transfer note may assist in providing continuity of nursing care when patients are transferred to another unit within the same hospital or to another hospital.

2. It is a means of communicating directions for out-patient care or follow-up when patients are discharged to their homes, to extended care facilities, or to nursing homes. In many instances, the patient and/or his family is given a copy of the discharge note for a summary of his nursing

117

problems (resolved and unresolved). This often provides motivation by showing the patient what his problems were, the progress he has made, and what he must do to make further progress. Also, written directions are more apt to be used than those given verbally during the confusing procedure of being discharged from a hospital.

3. The discharge note provides data for public health nursing referrals and can be attached to the referral written by the physician. This prevents the necessity of writing a separate nursing referral.

4. Writing the nursing discharge note requires that the nurse review the entire record. While doing this, she may see relationships and gain insights that were not evident to her at an earlier time. In a sense, the nurse must audit her own charting and may learn both her strengths and weaknesses, and what areas of her thought process and/or recording procedures need improvement. This provides valuable experience for the nurse who strives to learn from what she has done.

Since the actual need for the nursing discharge summary varies greatly from patient to patient, the details of the data included will also differ. For example, if one is writing a discharge summary to be used by public health nurses who will care for the patient in the home, detailed information about family members, their interaction, suggestions of ways to approach the patient, family, and others, may be included. However, this same information may be unnecessary for a patient being discharged who has no need for further nursing care at the particular time. The major areas where differences in detail occur will be those sections titled ''Plans'' and ''Other Recommendations.''

DIRECTIONS FOR WRITING THE NURSING DISCHARGE NOTE

1. Title of the note.
   Example: Nursing Discharge Note, or Nursing Transfer Note
2. Date and time the note is written.
   Example: 11-22-73 (1415)
3. Introductory information.
   This includes name, age, sex, marital status, number of hospital admissions, patient's reason for hospitalization, length of hospitalization (date of admission and date of discharge or transfer) and destination.
   Example: This is the *(number)* hospital admission for *(name)*, a *(age)*, *(marital status)*, *(sex)*, admitted *(date)* for *(reason for hospitalization)* and discharged *(date)* to *(destination)*.
4. Summary of each nursing problem.
   a. For each nursing problem, both active and resolved, include the problem number, problem title, date first noted (even if problem title has changed from original), and date resolved or notation that problem is still active.

118

Example:
   #1 Problem title—noted 11-5-73, resolved 11-9-73
   #2 Problem title—noted 11-5-73, active

b. If the problem has been resolved, no additional information needs to be included.

c. If the problem is active, include:
   1) *Subjective data:* Summarize subjective data including initial manifestations, important changes during hospitalization, and status at present time.
   2) *Objective data:* Summarize objective observations made initially and during hospitalization; quantitate observations whenever possible. *Example:* measurements of size of decubitus ulcer initially, during hospitalization (state whether size increased or decreased), and at the present time.
   3) *Assessment:* Summarize progress achieved (including subjective and objective findings), in managing problem and probable explanation for these findings. Note whether or not additional nursing care is needed. If so, include opinion of probable results if present plan of management is continued.
   4) *Plan:* If noted above that additional nursing care is required, record specific plan recommended for management of the particular nursing problem.

d. Repeat steps one through four for each active problem.

5. Other recommendations.

   Any other pertinent information or suggestions may be included in this section. *For example:*

a. Suggestions of ways to approach the patient and/or family.

b. Whether or not the patient will be assuming primary responsibility for his care. If not, note who will be assuming it. Include any knowledge of the relationship between this person and the patient.

c. Assessment of family's ability to care for patient after discharge. Consider necessary knowledge, equipment, supplies, time, other obligations (job, own family, and so on).

d. Knowledge of patient's feelings about accepting help from others, specifically from person responsible for his care.

e. Knowledge of feelings of the person responsible for patient's care.

6. Nurse's signature, identification of the unit where she may be reached, and the unit phone number.

DIRECTIONS FOR WRITING AN EXPIRATION NOTE

When a patient expires, a note is written basically similar to the nursing discharge or transfer note:

1. Title of the note: Expiration Note

2. Date and time the note is written.
   Example: 4-16-73 (1100)
3. Identification of each nursing problem which was unresolved at time of death. For each of these, include:
   a. Number and title of the problem.
   b. *Subjective data:* Summarize subjective data including initial manifestations, important changes during hospitalization, and status of the problem up to the time of death.
   c. *Objective data:* Summarize objective observations made initially and during hospitalization. Quantitate observations whenever possible.
   d. *Assessment:* Summarize progress achieved in managing problem and probable explanation for these findings.
4. Repeat steps a through d for each nursing problem active at the time the patient died.
5. *Plan:* This section would be included only if data indicates that the family would benefit from further nursing care. Data reflecting this need would be recorded in the discussion of the problems identified above. The plan for recommended nursing care and its purposes would be included here.
   Example: Plan to arrange for public health nursing referral to periodically check Mr. Brown's urine for sugar and acetone.
6. Nurse's signature.

REFERENCE

1.   Weed, Lawrence L.: *Medical Records, Medical Education, and Patient Care.* The Press of Case Western Reserve University, Cleveland, Year Book Medical Publishers, Inc., Chicago, 1969, p. 83.

10

THE NURSING PROCESS

Professional nursing practice requires collecting data in order to determine what the patient needs from nursing, making a plan to meet these needs, implementing the plan, modifying the plan as necessary in view of new data and evaluating the results of the plan on the basis of what happened to the patient or the family. These steps comprise what we refer to as the nursing process.

Nursing deals with the immediate day-to-day needs and problems of daily living—those activities which people ordinarily carry on for themselves. Therefore, it must provide protection, comfort, nurturance, maintenance, and promotion of healthy bodily functions and behavior. The nurse works within an intimate and often highly emotional context. She is concerned with people who need help coping with diverse medical and emotional problems.

Nurses work with many patients, all of whom present multiple problems. Thus, each nurse must make numerous complex decisions which greatly influence the patients for whom she is responsible. Because little systematic investigation has been conducted in clinical nursing practice, nurses and nursing students lack the security and comfort of a scientific rationale upon which to base these decisions. Examples of these decisions include:

1. When is a newly diagnosed diabetic patient ready to learn about his disease and what he must do to be able to live with it?
2. How can we best help a particular man to die comfortably and with dignity?
3. How can we best help this woman who is never free of pain?
4. How can we help a man admit that he is sick and accept the help he needs?
5. How can we help a woman begin to see health as more appealing than her sick role?
6. Which patients are most likely to experience skin breakdown?

Nursing is not an easy job, and requires the use of cognitive skills as well as the more common interpersonal and manual techniques which are better known and practiced by nurses. Furthermore, in view of the multitude and complexity of problems with which it deals, nursing must develop some systematic method of approaching and managing these problems.

This skit was written by nursing students to demonstrate why nurses need to collect data from patients:

Supervisor: And now, Miss Jones, will you tell us about the nursing care of this patient?

Nurse: This patient has been delightful to work with. He was very cooperative and undemanding. We really enjoyed having him on our floor.

Supervisor: That's very nice, Miss Jones . . . Now what were some of the *nursing problems* with this patient?

Nurse: Problems? . . . Let's see . . . Problems? . . . No, we didn't have any real problems with him that I can think of. As I said, he was very cooperative.

Supervisor: Certainly, you must have had *some* problems. The care involved with a newly diagnosed diabetic adolescent isn't easy. How much does he know about his diabetes?

Nurse: Oh, he *knows* about it, I'm sure . . . We've all been telling him about it.

Supervisor: Who has been telling him?

Nurse: Why, all of us . . . the nurses.

Supervisor: What have you told him?

Nurse: Well, actually, I haven't been working very closely with the actual teaching, but Miss Blake assures me that he knows everything he needs to know about diabetes.

Supervisor: Did anyone teach him to test his own urine and to keep accurate records?

Nurse: Miss Stone has been checking his urine; but she's off today. I don't know what she has been doing as far as teaching, but I imagine she has. She is very competent, you know.

Supervisor: I have spoken to you before, but perhaps it will help to go over it again. His urine records are incomplete. The doctor's order was for urine to be tested for sugar and acetone four times daily, before each meal and at bedtime. Accurate records are essential if the doctor is to regulate his insulin. Were these tests done four times a day?

Nurse: I'm sure that they were done, but you know how busy we get. Sometimes we just don't have time to record our results.

Supervisor: These things aren't discussed in your nursing progress notes; I've looked. How do you know that any teaching has actually be done?

Nurse: Why, the nurses have told me in report. We discuss everything in report.

Supervisor: How do you know that this patient learned anything if, indeed, any teaching took place?

Nurse: Why, I know! I know just from talking to him. He says that he knows all about diabetes. That's what he said!

Supervisor: Miss Jones, may I ask just what you *did* do for this patient?

Nurse: Why, we gave him three books to read, all explaining diabetes, hygiene, and diet.

Supervisor: Miss Jones, how well can your patient read?

Nurse: I don't really know. They were pretty simple books.

Supervisor: He can't read at all. He has had no formal education because he is supporting his family. Didn't you do a Nursing History on this patient?

Nurse: No. We just haven't had time. Now, Mrs. Green, are you criticizing how we cared for this patient?

Supervisor: Yes, I am criticizing your care, because you have no documentation that you did anything for this patient. You can't even tell me what you wanted to do for him.

Nurse: Mrs. Green, you know that we give patient-centered care in this hospital. Our first concern is the patient. Our intentions were good!

Supervisor: Yes, but good intentions by themselves, at best, result in patients surviving in spite of us.

How different would this exchange between the nurse and her supervisor have been if a Nursing History had been taken on this patient? According to Weed, accurate and complete information is essential to the management of patient care and that in the long run, it saves time and effort to gather it at the beginning of patient care, rather than try to improvise without it.[1]

How different would the dialogue have been if one nurse had been responsible for planning and evaluating the nursing care of this patient, and for documenting the plan and its results? This would have enabled everyone concerned to have access to the same information about the patient, his needs and nursing problems, the most up-to-date plan for meeting these needs and managing his problems, as well as the effect of the plan thus far. If all this information is recorded, no nurse need be placed in the position of Miss Jones to assume, guess, rationalize, and defend what the nurses responsible for the patient's care are doing.

If the system advocated in this manual had been utilized, the nurse responsible for the patient in the skit would have clearly stated a plan of what she wanted to do for and with this patient. We must *plan* and *state* precisely all nursing objectives in order that nursing care can be evaluated.

Since the only way to evaluate nursing care is to determine whether or not it makes a difference to the patient, the statement of nursing care objectives must be written in terms of the behavior the patient will demonstrate as a result of the nursing care he receives.

What the nurse accomplishes for and with patients must be measured in a systematic way and put into words that can be understood.[2] The results of nursing care can be observed and evaluated if the nurse defines the behavior the patient is expected to perform as a result of the nursing care he receives, the conditions under which the behavior is to occur, and the criteria of acceptable performance. However, these results must be recorded in order to be used by other health team members. If relayed verbally, valuable information which could be used to enhance the care of a particular patient, as well as the care of future patients with similar problems, will be lost forever. If proper records had been kept on the patient discussed above, Miss Jones would have had the results of the nurses' efforts available and would have been able to tell the supervisor precisely what was accomplished with and for the patient.

The use of this process of nursing practice requires collaboration among members of the health team. Experience has shown that when a nurse can present documented evidence of a patient's progress or failure to progress toward the desired objectives, other members of the health team are much more apt to listen to what she has to say. Had the problem-oriented system been utilized with the patient discussed in the skit, the dialogue between the staff nurse and the supervisor could have been one of true collaboration rather than a question–answer session resulting in the staff nurse becoming more and more defensive and the supervisor becoming more and more frustrated.

Current criteria of the Joint Commission on Accreditation of Hospitals requires that there be evidence of a nursing plan of care for every patient. Standard IV states:

There shall be evidence established that the nursing service provides safe, efficient, and therapeutically effective nursing care through the planning of each patient's care and effective implementation of the plans.[3]

In order to provide this evidence a written plan of nursing care must be part of each patient's permanent record.

The first stage of developing a clinical science in nursing consists of keeping records of professional clinical experiences. A review of many such patient records will provide the descriptive material necessary to develop categories of nursing problems, a language, predictive outcomes, and finally, a scientific rationale for practice. These records of nursing care will supply ideas and methods which practicing nurses and nursing students can react to, learn from, validate, or invalidate.[4] The Clinical Nursing

124

Tool described in this text, when used with the problem-oriented system, provides the means by which to organize the clinical practice of nursing.

REFERENCES

1. Weed, Lawrence L.: *Medical Records, Medical Education, and Patient Care*. The Press of Case Western Reserve University, Cleveland, Year Book Medical Publishers, Inc., Chicago, 1969, p. 58.
2. Smith, Dorothy M.: "Writing objectives as a nursing practice skill." *American Journal of Nursing* 71:320, 1971.
3. Porterfield, John D.: "Joint Commission on Accreditation of Hospitals," *American Journal of Nursing* 71:72, 1971.
4. Smith, Dorothy M.: "Is it too late?" *Nursing Clinics of North America*, W. B. Saunders Company, Philadelphia, 6:228, 1971.

11

PATIENT EXAMPLES

Addressograph Stamp	Nursing History

6-25-72 (1120)

I. Vital statistics: This is the second General Hospital admission for Mrs. Lorna Strong, a 46 year old woman from Lima, Florida.

II. Patient's understanding of illness: Patient had a constant, sharp pain in left front and side chest (under lowest rib) for 3 days. Pain was sharper at times (unpredictable); went to physician and was told she had a blood clot in her spleen or kidney. Sent to General Hospital for evaluation and treatment. Pain has not affected activities as went to physician and was sent here almost immediately. In 1963, had a cardiac catheterization which showed advanced valvular disease and surgery was advised. Refused surgery and was told her life expectancy was 6 months. Felt that God would allow her to live in order to bring up her children. In January, 1972, patient obtained a divorce after 23 years of marriage (stated husband was an "alcoholic"). Has been going through menopause for last 3 months (feels nervous and has irregular menstrual periods), another thing going on in her life at this time is that patient is trying to decide whether to put her lump sum divorce settlement into property as an investment.

III. Patient's expectations: Expects surgical removal of blood clot in spleen or kidney, and relief of pain during hospitalization. Expects nurses to give her medication. Did not expect to be put on I.V. medication (Heparin) or that question of heart surgery would be raised (which it was) early in admission procedure by physician.

127

IV. Brief social and cultural history: Divorced since January (see category II). Has 6 children, 4 of whom live at home, sometimes with patient in mobile home or with husband who lives ½ mile away. Youngest is 16 year old boy. Patient wanted to live by self most of time because of "menopause nerves." Finished 9th grade; has never worked outside home. Only concern is financial (hospital bill). Her children are the most significant persons to her.

V. Significant data in terms of:
A. Sleeping patterns: To bed by 2200; wakes and gets up at 0800. Twice a month watches late movie. No difficulty falling asleep and does not wake up during night. Watches TV ā sleep. Uses 1 pillow.
B. Eliminating patterns: B.M. q.d. p̄ breakfast. Last B.M. 6-25-72. Since pain started, has taken 2 bile salts tablets q.d. to reduce stomach edema and to move bowels. No problems ā this illness. States she does not know what maintains her bowel pattern except the habit of time. No difficulty c̄ voiding.
C. Breathing: No difficulty usually. Since present illness has trouble getting breath, especially when sharp pain is present. Keeps trying to get breath by panting. When this doesn't work, lies down and tries to calm herself by praying. This usually works; also helps when pain begins to subside. At present nose breathing, using thoracic muscles, breathing inaudible c̄ no signs of distress.
D. Eating and drinking patterns: Breakfast (0800) cereal or egg, toast, 1 cup coffee. No lunch except ice cream and cookie at 1200. Dinner (1700–1800) meat, vegetable, bread. Drinks 1300 cc. fluid daily, consisting of coffee, fruit juices, milk. Does not drink water. States she is "picky." Doesn't feel like eating; doesn't care for meat. Has a tendency to eat whatever is easiest to get, especially when children are c̄ father. Takes longer to eat since stroke. Had right sided stroke 2 years ago; affected swallowing and speech (since restored) and right arm and leg. Learned to use left hand for care and feeding. Will need someone to open cartons, butter bread, and put cream in coffee since has I.V. in left forearm for Heparin administration.
E. Skin integrity: Skin is yellowish, smooth, moist, and firm. Has reddish, raised mole-like lesions on front and back chest. Soft swelling 3 inches in diameter over right hip. Has had both of these for 10–12 years. Swelling hurts when lies on it. Has I.V. in left forearm; no swelling or redness at site. I.V. running as ordered. Uses body lotion (has c̄ her). Takes bath or shower ā bed (likes bath but shower easier). Shaves legs and underarms once/month. Has upper and lower dentures. Uses Efferdent (has c̄ her) p̄ dinner. Sleeps c̄ dentures in place. Usually needs

no help c̄ hygiene but c̄ I.V. in "good" arm may need help though she thinks she can manage.

F. Activity: Limps (aftermath of stroke). Doesn't get tired walking and no other effect observed. Right arm functional; can't use right hand except for large objects. Can't pick up small objects c̄ right hand. Can use eating implements c̄ right hand but very slowly and awkwardly. Has minimum "squeeze" power in right hand. Has learned to use left hand for all activities including writing. Has full R.O.M. in all joints except can't move right arm back any further than side. No prostheses.

G. Recreation: Watches TV, talks to neighbors, reads Bible (doesn't have c̄ her). Wants to watch 2 TV soap operas if possible.

H. Interpersonal and communicative patterns: Feels comfortable (at ease) in new situations and in meeting new people. Lying quietly on back, turned on side toward me once when talking about not wanting heart surgery. Answered all questions, volunteered information, spoke clearly and distinctly, stayed on subject. Asked questions about Heparin. Showed little emotion (facial expression did not change nor did body posture except as noted above when talking about pain, heart surgery, previous 6 months life expectancy, stroke, divorce).

I. Temperament: Gets angry when husband "drunk" against her wishes and when children smoke and drink (not doing what is "right according to the Bible"). Tells people what is "right" when angry. States that people know when she is angry because she tells them. Then said she doesn't really get angry, just doesn't like things that aren't "right."

J. Dependency and independency patterns: Likes to sew, crochet, and cook for self. Does housework for people who are ill. Others do housework for her when she is ill. States she has never had to ask for help, "people just do it." Doesn't know how she would ask for help or how she would feel since doesn't ask for help. States she's had no experience in working c̄ others.

K. Senses: Needs glasses (has c̄ her) for reading. No problems hearing. Left handed since stroke.

L. Menstrual patterns: Has menstruated q. 24–26 days for 5 days until 3 months ago. Has only menstruated once in 3 months for 3 days. States that physician told her she was starting menopause. No difficulty c̄ periods.

VI. Statement of that which makes the patient feel cared for: Bible, pictures of children when they were babies and children's gifts that she has kept are items which help patient feel secure. Neighbors doing housework for her makes her feel cared for.

Additional data: The following data was obtained when patient was asked if she had any questions or if she wanted to tell me anything else. At 0800 this morning, patient had an almost unbearable pain in left lower front chest and could not get breath. Kept trying to get breath and almost "blacked out." States she lay across bed and finally got better after 5 minutes. Was upset because no pain medication had been ordered for such attacks. (Physician has since ordered pain medication.) Says she kept "panting" to get breath. Also expressed concern that she had not received heart pill (digoxin) for the day. On checking found that next digoxin is due at 2200 and then tomorrow A.M. Patient advised of digoxin schedule. Stated she would refuse heart surgery, all she wanted was to get rid of blood clot and pain.

Lunch was served during this period. Validated that the only help patient needs is to have cartons opened, bread buttered, and cream put in coffee. Showed patient how to fill out menu and she can do this unassisted. Patient complained about I.V. saying that she felt tied to the bed and couldn't do for herself as she would like to.

G. Robbins, R.N.

#	Nursing Problems	Date	
		First Noted or Change of Title	Resolved
1.	Formation of emboli		
A.	Chest pain	6-25-72	
B.	Restricting effects of I.V. on independence	6-25-72	6-29-72
C.	Maintenance of I.V. patency	6-25-72	6-30-72
D.	Constipation	6-27-72	
E.	Vaginal bleeding	6-29-72	
2.	Worries		
A.	Lacks knowledge of medication and treatment schedule	6-25-72	
B.	Lacks financial resources	6-25-72	
C.	Doesn't want heart surgery	6-25-72	6-29-72
	Modified -- worries about surgery	6-29-72	
3.	Important to read Bible and watch T.V.	6-25-72	6-26-72
4.	Residual effect of stroke on right side	6-26-72	

6-25-72 (1430) Initial Plan

Problem #1A—Chest pain

Subjective data: Constant pain in lower front and side of chest below ribs. Has much sharper pain at times (unpredictable) which causes her to be unable to get deep breath. Pants in order to get breath; had one episode earlier today and almost "blacked out" during attack.

131

Objective data: Has advanced valvular disease c̄ almost certain mesenteric emboli; Morphine ordered P.R.N. for pain.

Assessment: Pain probably due to mesenteric emboli. May decrease c̄ Heparin administration which will decrease formation of new clots. Patient doesn't seem distressed c̄ constant pain, but perhaps a regular schedule of a mild analgesic will both serve to relax patient and reduce number of sharp pain attacks. Near black out may have been due to hyperventilation due to panting. Abdominal breathing instruction may be helpful.

Plan: Objective #1A—Sharp pain attacks will decrease in number.
1. Ask physician today about milder and regularly given analgesic
2. Instruct patient today about abdominal breathing—Show and have practice.
3. Ask patient to demonstrate abdominal breathing 6-26-72.

Problem #1B—Restricting effects of I.V. on independence
Subjective data: Feels tied to bed and unable to do for self as would like to.

Objective data: I.V. in left forearm, hanging from bed pole. Uses left hand for all activities since stroke 2 years ago. Unable to manipulate small objects c̄ right hand.

Assessment: I.V. put in before anyone knew patient left handed. (Wonder why she didn't ask that I.V. be put in right arm.) Will have I.V. for some time since medical plan is to give Heparin until prothrombin time is at a designated level (not definitely determined at this time), gradually reduce Heparin, give Coumadin while reducing Heparin, and discharge on Coumadin alone. Patient does not need to stay in bed.

Plan:
1. Obtain walking I.V. pole today and practice patient in using it safely.
2. Ask Occupational Therapy to see patient and devise eating utensils that will be easier for patient to use.
3. Place following directions on Kardex: At each meal, open cartons, put cream in coffee, and butter bread.
4. Will observe and help patient in personal hygiene activities 6-26-72 at 0830 to find what help she needs.

Problem #1C—Maintenance of I.V. patency
Subjective data: None
Objective data: I.V. running as ordered at keep-open rate.
Assessment: Need to guard against infection, infiltration, and bleeding.
Plan:
1. Will construct a flow sheet to be put on bedside chart for recording the following data:

a. Daily dressing change.

b. Condition of site q2h (bleeding, swelling, redness, and pain).

c. Rate of flow and amount infused q2h.

2. Will write following directions on Kardex:

a. Change dressing on I.V. site; clean site c̄ saline and apply Neosporin ointment q.d. at 0900 and note on flow sheet.

b. Check site for bleeding, swelling, redness, and pain q2h on odd hours and note observations on flow sheet.

c. Check rate of flow and amount infused q2h on odd hours and record on flow sheet.

Problem #2A—Lacks knowledge of medication/treatment schedule

Subjective data: Worried that hasn't had daily digoxin; didn't realize was going to be on Heparin or that heart surgery would be a possibility.

Objective data: None.

Assessment: Seems to be an immediate need or at least a focus for anxiety.

Plan:

1. Inform today of present medication and treatment schedule and reason for these.

2. Inform patient of changes as they occur.

3. Inform patient of diagnostic test schedule and supplement as necessary physician's explanation of such.

Problem #2B—Lacks finances

Subjective data: Concerned about hospital bill.

Objective data: None.

Assessment: Not enough data.

Plan: Will explore this c̄ patient on 6-26-72.

Problem #2C—Doesn't want heart surgery

Subjective data: Says she will refuse heart surgery.

Objective data: Refused heart surgery previously and has lived 9 years in spite of poor prognosis (6 months life expectancy).

Assessment: Not enough data. Know she refused surgery ā, feeling God would spare her to raise children. Don't know reason for this refusal.

Plan: Will explore this area c̄ patient on 6-26-72.

Problem #3—Important to read Bible and watch TV

Subjective data: Stated above.

Objective data: None.

Assessment: None.

Plan:

1. Obtain Bible from chaplain's office for patient today.

2. Ask patient if wishes to see hospital or community clergyman on 6-26-72.
3. Show patient TV room today and show her how to operate TV.

G. Robbins, R.N.

6-26-72 (1100) Nursing Progress Note

Problem #1A—Chest pain

Subjective data: "Breathing like you taught me helps me get good deep breaths." Has had codeine twice but can't tell yet if helps constant pain or not. Has not had another attack of sharp pain.

Objective data: New order for codeine 30 mg. p.o. q6h. Has had 2 doses. Using abdominal breathing as taught. Has not had P.R.N. morphine.

Assessment: Wonder if she really wants codeine even though she said she'd like to try it when I talked c̄ her about this yesterday.

Plan: Will continue to evaluate effects of codeine.

Problem #1B—Restricting effects of I.V. on independence

Subjective data: Likes walking I.V. pole; enables her to get around.

Objective data: O.T. consult. sent. O.T. will see patient this afternoon. Observed patient in personal hygiene activities. Found that she can and wants to manage (though slowly and awkwardly) except for washing back, buttocks, and back of thighs. Using walking I.V. pole and handling I.V. tubing correctly.

Plan: Will write following directions on Kardex: Assist patient c̄ bath by washing back, buttocks, and back of thighs.

Problem #1C—Maintenance of I.V. patency

Subjective data: Likes nurses checking I.V. Makes her feel safe.

Objective data: Flow sheet up to date; shows no problems.

Assessment: None.

Plan: Continue present plan.

Problem #2A—Lacks knowledge of medication/treatment schedule

Subjective data: Likes explanations; doesn't worry as much if knows what is going on.

Objective data: None.

Assessment: None.

Plan: Continue present plan.

Problem #2B—Lacks financial resources

Subjective data: Doesn't know how will pay hospital bill. Is getting welfare payments due to right sided disability (can't work). Has lump sum divorce settlement but doesn't want to use this since it's all she has and "there never will be any more." Thinking of buying property (to lease) so will have a little income. Angry at welfare worker in home town as she found out about settlement money in bank. Would like to work, perhaps get some training for a job, but welfare would not approve physical therapy so could strengthen right side.

Objective data: Patient did not gesture, alter body posture, or change facial expression in telling above. Spoke in monotone, but quickly and in jerks.

Assessment: This is a problem. Might be eligible for Vocational Rehabilitation funds (which she had when here for previous heart evaluation), but these funds depend on ability to work and she now has residual effects from stroke. Social security funds depend on total disability.

Plan:
1. Ask public health referral nurse to see patient and help c̄ paper work, contact welfare worker, and Vocational Rehabilitation people.
2. Add new problem #4—Residual effect of stroke on right side. Will ask Physical Therapy to see patient and evaluate whether something can be done to strengthen right side for possible job training.

Problem #2C—Doesn't want heart surgery.

Subjective data: Feels that can't burden children c̄ bills for this. Also feels she'll die from surgery. Feels that God spared her once and that she can't ask Him for more. Is willing to have cardiac catheterization scheduled for 8-30.

Objective data: Facial expression did not change during conversation. No gesture or other body movement except for reaching for my hand when saying she'd die from surgery.

Assessment: Hard to figure. Odd that she is willing to have cardiac catheterization if not willing to have surgery. Think finances important in this; really doesn't want to spend settlement money ($10,000) on hospital bills as will then have nothing. Physicians convinced of necessity of surgery. Wonder if she has been told that future strokes are a real possibility. Independence is important to her. Feel she is ambivalent and depressed, at the least, about making a decision.

Plan: Objective #2C—Patient will talk about feelings and thoughts related to surgery q.d.
1. Sit down and talk c̄ patient at least once daily about her feelings and thoughts related to surgery.
2. Tell patient that this time is specifically for above purpose.
3. Ask patient to identify pros and cons of having surgery.
4. Talk c̄ physician about stroke possibility as an angle of approach.
5. Ask physicians to advise me if they are going to speak c̄ patient about surgery at any time outside regular rounds so I can be present.

Problem # 3—Important to read Bible and watch TV
  Subjective data: Appreciates getting Bible; would like to see hospital chaplain. Glad to keep up c̄ TV soap operas. "Their problems are worse than mine."
  Objective data: None.
  Assessment: None.
  Plan:
  1. Ask chaplain to see patient.
  2. Discontinue as an active problem.

G. Robbins, R.N.

6-27-72 (0900) Nursing Progress Note
Problem #1A—Chest pain
  Subjective data: "Codeine makes me feel confused and dopey and doesn't help my pain." Thinks aspirin would be better when needs something. Is used to the constant pain; it's the unexpected sharp pain that "can't stand." Now knows "how to breathe better, which helps."
  Objective data: None.
  Assessment: Aspirin contraindicated as on anticoagulant Heparin.
  Plan:
  1. Ask physician to discontinue codeine and write P.R.N. order for Tylenol.
  2. Explain to patient why can't have aspirin.
  3. Tell patient to ask for Tylenol if needs it.
  4. Tell patient not to use aspirin when discharged on Coumadin, but to use Tylenol instead.

Additional Information
  Subjective data: Feels constipated; hasn't had B.M. for 2 days.
  Objective data: Taking codeine last 2 days.
  Assessment: I don't know if this is due to codeine, mesenteric emboli, inactivity, or worry.
  Plan: Add New Problem #1D—Constipation
  Objective #1D—Patient will have B.M. by noon on 6-28-72.
  1. Ask physician for MOM order stat and give.
  2. Request MOM order for P.R.N. h.s.
  3. Suggest to patient that she try to have B.M. at habitual time p̄ breakfast.
  4. Tell patient to walk length of hall q.i.d. (1000, 1400, 1800, 2200) using walking I.V. pole.
  5. Tell patient to try to drink 3 glasses water in addition to usual fluid intake.

Problem #2B—Lacks financial resources

Subjective data: Talked c̄ public health nurse; told what had to do to get financial help.

Objective data: Public health nurse's note indicates patient given application to complete for welfare disability. Will need letter from physician regarding disability and prognosis. Patient will need to take completed application and letter to local welfare office.

Assessment: None.

Plan: Help as needed c̄ application; make sure patient understands what she has to do.

Problem #2C—Doesn't want heart surgery

Subjective data: "I guess I have no choice. I'll have to have surgery because I don't want to be a burden on my children."

Objective data: Advised by physician that future strokes were almost inevitable and that she could be completely disabled and dependent. Patient asked about her chances of survival from surgery and was told that wouldn't know until p̄ cardiac catheterization. Asked no questions about surgical procedure.

Assessment: Feel that being a "burden" either financially or physically is unacceptable to patient. She can depersonalize getting help from welfare or nurses since this giving of help is their job. Will probably begin to accept surgery, intellectually at least.

Plan: No change.

Problem #4—Residual effect of stroke on right side

Subjective data: Physical therapist gave exercises to maintain present function of right side. Feels discouraged that nothing can be done to improve function so she can get a job.

Objective data: P.T. indicates that improvement is unlikely. Patient given leg, arm, and hand exercises to maintain present mobility. P.T. plans to give her a shoulder brace to be used when in bed to prevent contractures.

Assessment: Looks as if job is unlikely. Too many factors against (heart, right sided weakness, lack of training). Might be something to look into if makes good recovery from surgery. P.T. will follow while in hospital and give discharge instructions.

Plan: Objective #4—Patient will maintain present functioning of right arm, hand and leg.
1. Watch patient perform right arm, hand, and leg exercises b.i.d. (1000, 2000) per P.T. instruction sheet.
2. Point out in a matter of fact manner those things patient is able to do for self, such as "You did _____ today."

G. Robbins, R.N.

6-27-72 (1400) Nursing Progress Note
Problem #1B—Restricting effects of I.V. on independence
   Subjective data: Likes large eating implements.
   Objective data: Given above implements by O. T.
   Assessment: Above utensils help patient to be less awkward and slow in
      eating. Still needs help as indicated earlier c̄ opening cartons, putting
      cream in coffee, and buttering bread.
   Plan: Continue present plan of assistance c̄ meals.

                                                         G. Robbins, R.N.

6-28-72 (1300) Nursing Progress Note
Problem #1D—Constipation
   Subjective data: Bowels have not moved in spite of 2 doses (60 cc.)
      MOM and prune juice. Thinks prune juice on a regular basis might
      help. Very concerned that it is now 3 days s̄ B.M.
   Objective data: No. B.M. for 3 days.
   Assessment: Probably should have enema since she is concerned and
      since usual pattern is q.d.
   Plan: Ask physician for stat Fleets enema order and give stat.

                                                         G. Robbins, R.N.

6-28-72 (1500) Nursing Progress Note
Problem #1D—Constipation
   Subjective data: Feels much better now that bowels have moved.
   Objective data: Large amount of soft formed stool resulted from Fleets.
   Assessment: Since stool soft and formed and since excretion occurred
      immediately after enema, I don't know why patient couldn't move
      bowels.
   Plan: Modify Objective #1D—Patient will move bowels q.d. p̄ break-
      fast.
      1. Show patient how to check prune juice on menu.
      2. Tell patient to ask for MOM h.s. on days bowels haven't moved.
      3. Continue activity and fluid orders.

Problem #2A—Lacks knowledge of medication/treatment schedule
   Subjective data: None
   Objective data: To be started on Coumadin c̄ reduction in Heparin in
      A.M.
   Assessment: None
   Plan: Will explain this to patient this afternoon.

Problem #2B—Lacks financial resources
   Subjective data: None.
   Objective data: Patient filled out application for welfare c̄ help. Letter
      from physician cannot be obtained until discharge. Physician will send
      letter to patient. Note put on front of patient's chart to remind him.

138

Assessment: Wonder if she will follow through c̄ this. Could have filled out application herself, but waited for me to help her. "Forgot" to ask physician for letter until reminded twice.

Plan: Will ask public health referral nurse to send a public health referral to patient's local county health department to provide further help c̄ seeking financial assistance, to make sure physician's letter arrives, to check on whether patient taking Coumadin as ordered, and getting blood counts as ordered. Public health nurse might also help patient explore feelings about returning for cardiac catheterization and heart surgery. Physician has agreed to public health referral for above reasons.

G. Robbins, R.N.

6-29-72 (0900) Nursing Progress Note
Problem #1A—Chest pain

Subjective data: Pain which patient had when admitted has gradually decreased, but at 0800 had pain in right upper chest on breathing. Thinks has cold from air conditioner. Refused Tylenol; doesn't like to take pain medication.

Objective data: X-rays negative for congestion or pulmonary emboli. No rise in temperature or pulse; no change in blood pressure. No cough.

Assessment: Physicians think perhaps a mild pleurisy, but not sure. Since patient refuses medication, wonder if old fashioned binder will help.

Plan: Will get straight binder and put on patient this A.M.

Problem #1C—Maintenance of I.V. patency

Subjective data: Glad that I.V. now in right arm.

Objective data: I.V. infiltrated at 0400; site reported to be slightly red, swollen, and painful. New I.V. put in right forearm. Original site no longer red, swollen or painful, probably due to application of heat and relatively short duration of infiltration (I.V. checked at 0315 and was OK).

Assessment: Wonder just how often I.V. should be checked to prevent infiltration. Apparently no clues at 0315 to indicate impending infiltration. This needs study.

Plan: Continue present plan of checking; Problem #1B no longer an active problem as I.V. no longer in left arm and patient has walking I.V. pole. Discontinue orders for Problem #1B. Problem resolved.

Problem #2B—Lacks financial resources

Subjective data: Feels that public health nurse will be helpful to her.

Objective data: Public health referral sent; to follow patient at home for further exploration of financial help needed, checking on medications,

139

exploration of feelings related to cardiac catheterization and heart surgery, and arranging transportation for blood work if necessary.

Assessment: Believe that patient can and will use help from public health nurse.

Plan: Nothing further at this time.

Problem #2C—Doesn't want heart surgery

Subjective data: Will have heart surgery if some way can be found to pay for it. More afraid of being "like a vegetable from a stroke" than of surgery or death. Said chaplain helped her to decide.

Objective data: Again very little facial expression or bodily movement during conversation.

Assessment: Hard to know what thinking or feeling, but is saying the "right" words.

Plan: Will continue to listen to patient as she talks about surgery. Modify problem title to "Worries about surgery," as no longer refusing surgery.

G. Robbins, R.N.

6-29-72 (1800) Nursing Progress Note

Problem #1A—Chest pain

Subjective data: Binder "feels good; it doesn't hurt as much to breath." Coughing, still thinks has cold.

Objective data: No fever. Cough dry, seems to be from throat or trachea. No sputum.

Assessment: None.

Plan: Continue present plan.

Additional Information

Subjective data: Vaginal bleeding. Menstrual periods have been irregular.

Objective data: Discharge is dark blood; has used 1 pad in 4 hours; moderate bleeding.

Assessment: In view of anticoagulants, need to watch for hemorrhage.

Plan:
1. Ask patient to call nurse when changes pads.
2. Write following directions on Kardex:
   a. Patient will call nurse when wishes to change pads.
   b. Check pads for excessive soaking c̄ bright blood and for steady dripping from vagina.
   c. Record condition of pad and time on flow sheet at bedside.
3. Add New Problem #1E—Vaginal bleeding, to problem list.

G. Robbins, R.N.

6-30-72 (1000) Nursing Progress Note
Problem #1A—Chest pain
  Subjective data: Pain disappeared during night. Thinks reason is shutting
    off air conditioner. Doesn't need.binder anymore. No recurrence of
    admission pain.
  Objective data: None.
  Assessment: None.
  Plan: Ask patient to let us know if she has any kind of pain again.

Problem #1C—Maintenance of I.V. patency
  Subjective data: Glad to have I.V. out.
  Objective data: I.V. removed at 0900; patient now only on Coumadin.
  Assessment: None.
  Plan: Problem #1C no longer an active problem; discontinue all related
    orders. Problem resolved.

Problem #1D—Constipation
  Subjective data: B.M. p̄ breakfast 6-29-72 and 6-30-72. Feels prune juice
    is helping.
  Objective data: None.
  Assessment: For whatever reason, patient now back on usual schedule.
    Has P.R.N. order for laxative if desired, but seems unnecessary.
  Plan: Continue present plan.

Problem #2A—Lacks knowledge of medication/treatment schedule
  Subjective data: None.
  Objective data: To be discharged in A.M. on Coumadin and weekly
    prothrombin count at local physician's office.
  Assessment: None.
  Plan: Will help patient make out schedule for taking and recording
    medication.
                                                    G. Robbins, R.N.

6-30-72 (1500) Nursing Progress Note
Problem #1E—Vaginal bleeding
  Subjective data: Has used same number pads used during last menstrual
    period.
  Objective data: No report of heavy, bright bleeding. Flow almost
    stopped; hardly needs pad.
  Assessment: Probably menstrual period, although irregular. Physician
    concurs.
  Plan: Ask public health nurse to check at home.
                                                    G. Robbins, R.N.

7-1-72 (1300) Nursing Discharge Note

This was the 2nd General Hospital admission for Lorna Strong, a 46 year old divorced woman, admitted 6-25-72 for lower chest pain and "blood clots" and discharged to home 7-1-72 to be followed by local physician and public health department. To return 8-30-72 for cardiac catheterization and will then be scheduled for heart surgery for advanced valvular disease c̄ multiple emboli formation.

Problems	Noted	Resolved/Active
1. Formation of emboli		
A. Chest pain	6-25-72	Active
B. Restricting effects of I.V. on independence	6-25-72	Resolved 6-29-72
C. Maintenance of I.V. patency	6-25-72	Resolved 6-30-72
D. Constipation	6-27-72	Active
E. Vaginal bleeding	6-29-72	Active
2. Worries		
A. Lacks knowledge of medication and treatment schedule	6-25-72	Active
B. Lacks financial resources	6-25-72	Active
C. Doesn't want heart surgery	6-25-72	Resolved 6-29-72
Modified to:		
Worries about surgery	6-29-72	Active
3. Important to read Bible and watch TV	6-25-72	Resolved 6-26-72
4. Residual effect of stroke on right side	6-26-72	Active

Problem #1A—Chest pain

Subjective data: On admission had constant pain in lower front and side chest below ribs. Had sharper pain at times which made her unable to get breath. For 2 days had pain in chest which patient felt was a cold. Gradual decrease in complaints of pain until reports no pain at present time.

Objective data: Had codeine and morphine ordered for pain. Took codeine for 2 days. Felt it made her "dopey and confused" and that it didn't help pain. Wanted aspirin. Tylenol ordered as aspirin contraindicated by anticoagulant. Dislikes taking pain medication of any kind. Patient taught to abdominal breathe which helped during episodes of sharp pain, prevented hyperventilation and feeling of "blacking out." Binder used which patient thought helpful when had pain in chest and dry cough seemingly related to mild pleurisy.

Assessment: Knows to report reappearance of pain to physician and not take aspirin while on Coumadin. If pain due to clots, anticoagulation should prevent new emboli formation and thus may have no further pain.

Plan: Check for reappearance of pain, especially sharper chest pain.

Problem #1D—Constipation
    Subjective data: One episode of constipation (no B.M. for 3 days). Now has B.M. according to usual pattern.

    Objective data: Constipation not relieved by MOM; given Fleets enema once. Problem relieved and pattern maintained c̄ prune juice and attempting to have B.M. at usual time p̄ breakfast.

    Assessment: Problem could have been due to mesenteric emboli and reappearance might be a clue to further abdominal clot formation. However could also have been due to worries and reduced activity. Patient knows to report recurrence.

    Plan: Inquire about recurrence of constipation and remind patient to report.

Problem #1E—Vaginal bleeding
    Subjective data: Irregular menstrual periods for past 3 months (only 1 period in 3 months). Says starting menopause.

    Objective data: Vaginal bleeding began 6-29-72. Almost stopped by discharge 7-1-72.

    Assessment: Appears to be menstrual period, but should be checked as on anticoagulant and possibility of hemorrhage exists.

    Plan:
    1. Inquire about vaginal bleeding.
    2. Remind patient to report bleeding.
    3. Tell patient to record number of peri-pads required in particular length of time.

Problem #2A—Lacks knowledge of medication/treatment schedule
    Subjective data: Understands how to take and record Coumadin, side effects to watch for, and precautions to take while using anticoagulants (no aspirin, careful not to fall or bump self, etc.).

    Objective data: To go to local physician for weekly prothrombin count.

    Assessment: Believe patient will take medication as ordered. May need transportation to physician's office for blood work.

    Plan:
    1. Ask if further questions.
    2. Inquire about how patient plans on getting to physician's office.

Problem #2B—Lacks financial resources
    Subjective data: Worried about finances. Only money is lump sum divorce settlement which she's not willing to spend on surgery or hospital bill as it's all she has or will have.

Objective data: Has filled out application for financial aid. Will receive physician's letter that is needed within the week. Knows that these 2 documents must be taken to local welfare office.

Assessment: May need transportation and encouragement to follow through with obtaining financial aid. Think she will do it if encouraged (such as helping to fill out forms, reminding her to do it, arranging transportation). May have problem obtaining assistance as has some money. May need to sign this money over to children in order to qualify for assistance, but am not sure she will do this. Likes to talk c̄ clergyman ā making major decisions.

Plan:
1. Ask if has received physician's letter.
2. Ask how plans to get to local welfare office.
3. Inquire about status of problem when seeing patient.

Problem #2C—Worries about heart surgery

Subjective data: Refused heart surgery at first, partly because of financial reasons and partly because of fear of dying. Presently concerned about being "a vegetable," incapacitated if has another stroke.

Objective data: Told that s̄ surgery, inevitable stroke might cause her to be totally incapacitated.

Assessment: Seems to be more afraid of being burden to children and being incapacitated than afraid of surgery itself. Made decision to have surgery (if can obtain financial aid) p̄ talking c̄ chaplain. Still not sure we know whole story of how patient feels or what she is thinking.

Plan: Talk c̄ patient about feelings and thoughts related to having surgery and cardiac catheterization.

Problem #4—Residual effect of stroke on right side

Subjective data: Discouraged c̄ report from P.T. that no improvement possible.

Objective data: Limited use of right hand (can use only to handle large objects). Limited R.O.M. in right arm (unable to rotate or move beyond side) and limps.

Assessment: P.T. feels that no improvement possible, but that maintenance of present status is important. (Thus far this status has been maintained.) Given exercises to maintain status and shoulder brace to prevent contractures, to be used while in bed.

Plan:
1. Patient is to perform exercises according to instruction sheet (which she has) t.i.d.
2. Ask patient to perform exercises during visit.

3. Any suggestions or resources for job training that can be made in light of the above might be a morale booster to patient as she says she wants to work.

G. Robbins, R.N.
General Hospital
Medical Unit
Phone: 635-3292

2-19-73 (1500)

I. Vital statistics: 1st General Hospital admission for John Roberts, a 30 year old single man from Springer, Florida.

II. Patient's understanding of illness: Says he had a "pounding" left frontal headache 2 weeks ago beginning about 1000 and lasting until 1400. After 2nd day of this, went to physician who told patient he had high blood pressure (300/200). Admitted to local hospital. Given medication in hospital for B.P. and headache (doesn't know name of medication). Hasn't had headache since 3rd day of local hospital stay. Local physician said kidneys had only 5% function. Sent to General Hospital for evaluation of kidney problem and continued treatment of high B.P. B.P. now 130/92. Patient had not noticed decrease in urinary output; was surprised to find he had kidney trouble. First time had headache was at work, by himself, fixing a swing. Only effect on life is that has had to be in hospital and has missed work.

III. Patient's expectations: Expects tests (X-rays) to find out how well kidneys are working and to increase fluid intake from 500 cc. to 2000 cc. to see if kidneys can put out more. Expects to "get well" (have no more headaches). Expects nurses to watch his I and O (he can record this himself) and report to physicians q.d.

IV. Brief social and cultural history: Foreman at Springer Recreation Dept. Puts up and maintains equipment. Graduated from high school. Has mother, father, and 7 siblings who all live in another city. Lives c̄ aunt. Most significant person is mother. Has no concerns about family, job, or finances at this time.

V. Significant data in terms of:
   A. Sleeping patterns: Retires 2300; wakes and gets up 0500. Says prayers h.s. No problem getting to sleep or staying asleep. Uses 1 pillow.
   B. Eliminating patterns: B.M. t.i.d. at no particular time; last B.M. this A.M. Uses no aids and perceives nothing (diet, fluid, exercise) as maintenance measures. No problems c̄ B.M. or voiding. Reports no blood in urine, burning or increased frequency. I and O as recorded in other hospital for 2 days (patient has I and O record):

| 2-17-73 | Intake = | 660 cc. | Output = | 350 cc. |
| 2-18-73 | Intake = | 2030 cc. | Output = | 1150 cc. |

146

As of 1500 today, intake 1300 cc., output 250 cc. Patient demonstrated ability to keep I and O record accurately.

C. Breathing: Reports no problem. Rate 20/minute. Nose breathing, respirations quiet $\bar{s}$ flaring nostrils. No supra or subclavicular retractions. Smokes less than 1 pack/day.

D. Eating and drinking patterns: Breakfast (0600) toast, eggs, coffee. Lunch (1200) sandwich, cookies, soda. Supper (1800) meat, rice, vegetable, tea. Drinks 2 qts. fluid/day. Likes all juices. No problems $\bar{c}$ nausea, vomiting, or teeth interfering $\bar{c}$ eating. Knows that he is now on 40 Gm. protein, 2 Gm. sodium, 1800 calorie diet $\bar{c}$ 2000 cc. fluid intake, but doesn't understand diet. Has no food dislikes or religious restrictions. Present wt. is 86.0 Kg.

E. Skin integrity: Skin smooth, dry, brown, firm. No redness or darkness over bony prominences. Applies lotion to hands, face, and legs q.d.; feels this keeps skin less dry. Has hospital lotion to use. Takes tub bath q.d. at 1900; shaves q.d. at 0600. Now cannot see reflection clearly in mirror (blurred vision). Will need help shaving. Brushes teeth b.i.d. at 0600 and 1900; has brush and paste here. Needs no assistance $\bar{c}$ hygiene except that needs to be shaved until vision clears up.

F. Activity: No problems observed $\bar{c}$ walking; gait smooth, even, about 2 steps/second. Observed to have full R.O.M. in all joints. Requires no assistance. No prostheses.

G. Recreation: Fishing, dancing, playing baseball, basketball.

H. Interpersonal and communicative patterns: Feels "fine" in new situations and $\bar{c}$ people he doesn't know. Helps if others introduce themselves. Feels he can talk $\bar{c}$ anyone. Sat on chair during interview, scratched head 2–3 times, looked at me, held hands folded in lap. Answered all questions, spoke clearly and distinctly, stayed on topic, asked questions for clarification, volunteered information about I and O records and how he kept these.

I. Temperament: Reports that he can think of nothing that makes him angry, upset, or irritated. Says that headache did upset him because couldn't work. Thinks if he ever did get angry, he would tell the person, just as he went to the doctor about headache. Feels his religion keeps him free of anger.

J. Dependency and independency patterns: Prefers to do all his own hygiene activities, but is willing to let someone else shave him until can see adequately. Likes others to do his laundry. Cooks for others, takes meals to sick people. Asks directly for what needs (asked for help $\bar{c}$ shaving). He and fellow workers help each other to keep recreation area a

147

"nice, safe" place for children. Feels "thankful" when asking for and getting help, and when helping others.

K. Senses: Blind in left eye from childhood accident. Has had no effect on life except that sometimes worries about losing sight in other eye. As of this A.M. has "blurred vision." Cannot see to read or shave. Can see to mark intake on his own record. (Writes in time and amount in cc. Knows equivalents for ordinary hospital utensils.) Can see to move around room. No hearing problem. Right handed.

VI. Statement of that which helps patient feel cared for: Feels cared for when aunt does things for him (washes, irons, and cooks). Feels secure when has wallet c̄ him or knows where it is. (Has c̄ him now though most of money, for which he has a receipt, is in hospital safe.) Religion also helpful in making patient feel secure.

M. Hill, R.N.

#	Nursing Problems	Date	
		First Noted or Change of Title	Resolved
1.	Control of hypertension	2-19-73	
2.	Reduced kidney function	2-19-73	
A.	Diet restriction	2-19-73	2-23-73
B.	Intake - Output balance	2-19-73	2-22-73
3.	Blurred vision	2-19-73	2-22-73
A.	Dizziness	2-20-73	2-21-73
4.	Religion important to patient	2-19-73	2-20-73
5.			

2-19-73 (1700) Initial Plan

Problem #1—Control of hypertension

Subjective data: Expects to have B.P. lowered so will not have headaches. No headache for 8 days.

Objective data: B.P. decreased from reported 300/200 on initial visit to local physician to 130/92 on admission. Hypertensive drug therapy started at other hospital being continued here. Medical order is for supine and standing B.P. q6h in left arm c̄ the objective of a diastolic pressure of 90. Medical diagnosis of probable malignant hypertension c̄ chronic renal failure.

149

Assessment: Control of hypertension by drug therapy requires accurate taking and monitoring of B.P.

Plan:

1. Inform patient that B.P. will be taken lying and standing in left arm at 0600, 1200, 1800, and 2400.
2. Will place B.P. flow sheet marked to record above on bedside chart; ask shift team leader to check to see that procedure is followed and to report increase or decrease of 15 mm. or more in either diastolic or systolic pressure in any 6 hour period.

Problem #2—Reduced kidney function

Subjective data: Told kidneys had only 5% function; hadn't realized anything wrong c̄ kidneys.

Objective data: Chronic renal failure.

Assessment: None, insufficient data.

Plan: None.

Problem #2A—Diet restriction

Subjective data: Knows he's on a diet reduced in protein, sodium, and calories. Does not understand diet in relation to what foods and how much he's allowed. Says he's satisfied c̄ foods he's been getting on diet.

Objective data: Is on 40 Gm. protein, 2 Gm. sodium, 1800 calorie diet. Medical plan is to change diet in 2–3 days to 40 Gm. protein, 1800 calories, and unrestricted sodium.

Assessment: Better to wait until diet plan stable for discharge ā beginning teaching so as not to confuse patient c̄ different instructions.

Plan: Will request dietary consult for patient when diet plan stabilized.

Problem #2B—Intake-output balance

Subjective data: Says he is getting enough to drink. In other hospital, patient measured and recorded intake and nurses measured output which patient recorded.

Objective data: Patient demonstrated knowledge of the number of cc./ fluid containers. Demonstrated ability to record kind and amount of fluid in spite of blurred vision. Present fluid order is for 2000 cc./24 hours. Present wt. is 86.0 Kg.

Assessment: With medical plan to increase both fluid and sodium intake so as to increase blood volume and perfuse kidneys, accurate I and O records are essential to evaluate plan. Wt. gain expected, but hope that it will be slow. Important that patient gets all fluids he is allowed.

Plan:

1. Supervise patient today to insure his understanding and accuracy in measuring and recording intake and recording output.
2. Inform patient that he must use urinal and should ask nurse to measure output.

3. Plan c̄ patient a 24 hour fluid plan for intake of 2000 cc. and post this plan at bedside.
4. Will write following objective and orders in Kardex.
   Objective #2B—Patient will drink 2000 cc./24 hours.
   a. Team leader check I and O record at end of shift to see if intake planned for shift has been achieved.
   b. If not achieved, plan c̄ patient to make up deficit during next shift and advise next shift team leader.

Problem #3—Blurred vision
Subjective data: Unable to shave because can't see reflection clearly in mirror. Unable to see to read.
Objective data: Able to record I and O, see large objects, walk s̄ difficulty, and play cards c̄ other patients.
Assessment: Not sure whether blurred vision due to decrease in B.P. or to drugs. Patient concerned as already blind in one eye and now can't see to shave. Physicians feel this is a temporary problem.
Plan:
1. Will explain to patient today that physician feels this is a temporary problem and that it will go away, that someone will shave him and read his menu to him.
2. Will write following orders on Kardex:
   a. Shave patient q.d. at 0900 since he cannot see to shave self.
   b. Call dietary to have dietary aide read menu to patient so that he can make food choices.

Problem #4—Religion important to patient
Subjective data: Says prayers h.s., religion keeps him from getting angry and makes him feel secure.
Objective data: None.
Assessment: None.
Plan: Tell patient about religious resources available to him at General Hospital and in the community.

M. Hill, R.N.

2-20-73 (1000) Nursing Progress Note
Problem #1—Control of hypertension
Subjective data: Stated B.P. being taken per directions.
Objective data: Range of B.P. standing is 120/92 to 124/96. Range supine is 110/70 to 118/90.
Assessment: None.
Plan: Continue present plan.

Problem #2—Reduced kidney function
Subjective data: Says he is to have renal arteriogram on 2-22 and that he understands the procedure.

151

Objective data: Renal arteriogram ordered c̄ necessary prep orders. Physician's note indicates test explained to patient. Medical plan is to work patient up for hemodialysis and future kidney transplant.

Assessment: Feel it is premature to discuss dialysis and transplant c̄ patient at this time.

Plan:
1. Will talk c̄ patient today about procedure to see if he has any questions.
2. Remind patient today and tomorrow he is to be N.P.O. p̄ midnight on 2-21-73.

Problem #2B—Intake-output balance

Subjective data: Likes keeping own records; feels he's helping himself.

Objective data: Intake = 1595 cc. and output = 475 cc. on 2-19-73. Wt. increase from 86.0 Kg. to 86.1 Kg.

Assessment: Wt. increase insignificant at this time.

Plan: Continue present plan.

Problem #3—Blurred vision

Subjective data: Still can't see self clearly in mirror or see to read. Was shaved by assistant and menu read to him. Stated felt "dizzy" when got up at 0730. Room spinning sometimes from left to right and sometimes right to left c̄ no predictability. Said he got up slowly; not dizzy when supine.

Objective data: Walked c̄ feet wide apart, weaving from side to side, hanging onto bed or wall. No nystagmus noted. B.P. supine = 120/96, standing = 118/80.

Assessment: Appears that dizziness and blurred vision are transient and probably due to drug therapy.

Plan:
1. Continue present plan c̄ shaving and reading menu.
2. Add Problem #3A—Dizziness.
   a. Instruct patient immediately to walk only c̄ assistance as long as he is dizzy.
   b. Explain to patient possible cause and expected transient nature of problem.
   c. Note on Kardex that patient is to walk only c̄ assistance because of dizziness.
   d. Assist patient to get up slowly as follows:
      1. Roll up head of bed to 90° and have patient sit up in bed 2–3 minutes.
      2. Sit on side of bed and dangle 5 minutes.
      3. Stand at side of bed until steady.
      4. Then walk.

152

Problem #4—Religion important to patient
Subjective data: Feels he won't be here long enough to use religious resources in hospital. Was glad to know they are available.
Objective data: None.
Assessment: None.
Plan: Discontinue as active problem.

M. Hill, R.N.

2-20-73 (1700) Nursing Progress Note
Problem #2—Reduced kidney function
Subjective data: Understands arteriogram procedure.
Objective data: Explained what physician would do and what to expect before, during, and after procedure, as well as what is expected of him. No questions.
Assessment: Accurate explanation; apparent adequate understanding.
Plan:
1. Continue asking patient if he has any questions.
2. Plan to be c̄ patient ā he leaves for procedure.

Problem #3A—Dizziness
Subjective data: Still dizzy when stands.
Objective data: Walking the same as in A.M. Getting up according to procedure and only c̄ help.
Assessment: None.
Plan: Continue above.

M. Hill, R.N.

2-21-73 (0900) Nursing Progress Note
Problem #2A—Diet restriction
Subjective data: None.
Objective data: Diet order changed to 40 Gm. protein, 1500 calories, unrestricted salt.
Assessment: Patient needs instruction about diet now since this is his discharge diet.
Plan: Dietary consult. c̄ follow up.

Problem #2B—Intake-output balance
Subjective data: States no problem.
Objective data: No wt. gain; intake = 1090 cc. on 2-20-73 c̄ output of 550 cc. New order to force fluids to 3000 cc./day.
Assessment: Has not been getting required amount and now amount increased. May be problem to get intake of 3000 cc., especially as will be N.P.O. for arteriogram tomorrow.
Plan: Modify Objective #2B to: Patient will drink 3000 cc./24 hours. Will plan new fluid plan c̄ patient, post same and discuss with team leader.

Problem #3—Blurred vision
Subjective data: Can see to shave today, but still can't see to read.
Objective data: Shaved self; menu read to patient.
Assessment: Problem apparently resolving.
Plan:
1. Discontinue order for shaving patient.
2. Continue to read menu to patient.

Problem #3A—Dizziness
Subjective data: Dizziness disappeared during night.
Objective data: Gait has returned to status on admission.
Assessment: Transient nature of dizziness seems validated.
Plan:
1. Discontinue order for assisting patient to walk.
2. Tell patient to continue getting up slowly and to report any recurrence of dizziness to nurse.
3. Remind patient that if dizzy to walk only c̄ help.
4. Discontinue as active problem.

M. Hill, R.N.

2-22-73 (0800) Nursing Progress Note
Problem #1—Control of hypertension
Subjective data: None.
Objective data: B.P. within expected range and stabilized. Since 2-20-73 range supine = 120–124/92–96; standing = 110–118/70–90.
Assessment: Possibily B.P. taking could be decreased to b.i.d. p̄ today. Will have frequent vital sign monitoring today due to arteriogram.
Plan: Will ask physician about this.

Problem #2—Reduced kidney function
Subjective data: Will be glad when arteriogram finished.
Objective data: Has followed pretest orders.
Assessment: Doesn't seem upset, would just like to have procedure over with.
Plan: Will go c̄ patient to X-ray; will not stay, but will see him when returns from arteriogram.

Problem #2A—Diet restriction
Subjective data: Talked c̄ dietician and given list of foods allowed to eat. Dietician to return 2-23-73 to answer any questions.
Objective data: Dietician's note confirms the above. She says it's important to stress diet as a major part of patient's treatment while waiting for kidney transplant. Patient did not mention being told this.
Assessment: Wonder if patient understands importance of diet in relation to illness.

Plan:
1. Talk c̄ patient tomorrow and make sure he understands diet and its major treatment effects.
2. Objective #2A—Patient will write 2 sample menus for each meal by noon on 2-23-73.
   a. Ask patient to write out sample daily diets based on foods he likes and that he is allowed to have.
   b. Review c̄ dietician to make sure diets are within restrictions.

Problem #2B—Intake-output balance
Subjective data: None.
Objective data: Intake on 2-21-73 = 2850 cc., output = 650 cc. Wt. gain of 0.1 Kg.
Assessment: Due to arteriogram, patient will probably not be able to get 3000 cc. fluid today. Talked c̄ physicain who plans to change fluid order to ad lib. since patient gaining wt. slowly and showing no signs of edema or congestive heart failure. Patient usually drinks 2000 cc./day at home which physician says is sufficient now.
Plan:
1. Tell patient to try to drink the amount of fluid he usually drinks at home.
2. Discontinue Problem #2B as an active problem as well as related objective and orders for fluid plan and recording I and O.

Problem #3—Blurred vision
Subjective data: Able to shave self and read, now.
Objective data: Read from magazine to demonstrate ability to see.
Assessment: Problem resolved.
Plan: None. Discontinue related orders.

M. Hill, R.N.

2-22-73 (1500) Nursing Progress Note
Problem #2—Reduced kidney function
Subjective data: Procedure was just as expected except that didn't realize how hard it would be to lie still as long as was necessary. No pain at site, but back hurts.
Objective data: Returned from X-ray 1300. Vital signs stable; B.P. now 140/96 supine; prearteriogram B.P. 110/86. Arteriogram site (right groin) shows no bleeding or swelling. Right and left legs same temperature to touch. Femoral pulses equal in strength and rate bilaterally. Medical order for bed rest until 1000 2-23-73.
Assessment: Patient will have to stay in bed; not used to this. Perhaps back rubs will help.
Plan:
1. Will rub patient's back ā leaving.
2. Ask nursing assistants to rub back h.s. and during night if awakens.

Problem #1—Control of hypertension
Subjective data: Feels no differently from increased B.P.
Objective data: See note above for Problem #2.
Assessment: Increased B.P. may be due to arteriogram but more likely due to missed dosage of Aldomet while in X-ray and decrease of Aldomet by ½ this A.M. per medical order.
Plan:
  1. Change B.P. order to only supine taking until 1000 on 2-23-73.
  2. Discuss c̄ team leader about possibility for further increase in B.P.
M. Hill, R.N.

2-23-73 (0800) Nursing Progress Note
Problem #1—Control of hypertension
Subjective data: None.
Objective data: B.P. ranging from 140–160/100–110. Aldomet increased to original dosage.
Assessment: In view of B.P. increase and fact that medication is not yet regulated, will not ask for B.P. taking to be reduced to b.i.d. until diastolic pressure down to 90 mm. again and medication is regulated.
Plan:.None.
M. Hill, R.N.

2-23-73 (1400) Nursing Progress Note
Problem #2—Reduced kidney function
Subjective data: "I'm going to have a shunt put in so my blood can be cleaned out while I'm waiting for a new kidney." Will go home day p̄ shunt put in.
Objective data: Shunt ordered for 2-25-73. Physician has instructed patient about procedure.
Assessment: None.
Plan: Talk c̄ patient about shunt and answer any questions he may have.

Problem #2A—Restricted diet
Subjective data: Understands diet, now. Says making out diet plans really helped. Saw dietician today and she said sample diets were fine; also said diet is as important as my medicine.
Objective data: Dietary progress note confirms what patient reports.
Assessment: Patient seems to understand diet and is able to select foods in accordance c̄ restrictions.
Plan: Problem resolved; discontinue related objective and orders.
M. Hill, R.N.

2-24-73 (1100) Nursing Progress Note
Problem #1—Control of hypertension
Subjective data: None.
Objective data: B.P. seems stabilized at 130–136/90–94 supine and

156

120–124/88–90 standing. Medical order changed to B.P. supine or sitting b.i.d. To be discharged on present dose of Aldomet.

Assessment: Important to make sure patient understands about medication. Better to do this now rather than hurried instructions just ā discharge.

Plan:
1. Ask physician for prescription today so this can be taken care of and thus avoid waiting at discharge.
2. Help patient plan medication schedule around his usual daily schedule.

Problem #2—Reduced kidney function
Subjective data: None.
Objective data: Able to explain shunt procedure.
Assessment: None.
Plan: Continue to talk c̄ patient about shunt. Begin to inquire about his thoughts related to dialysis and future transplant.

M. Hill, R.N.

2-25-73 (1000) Nursing Progress Note
Problem #1—Control of hypertension
Subjective data: None.
Objective data: Shunt being put in left wrist this A.M.
Assessment: Necessary to institute measures to keep shunt working.
Plan:
1. Post sign at head of bed stating that no blood be drawn from left arm and no B.P. be taken in left arm.
2. Note in Kardex to take B.P. in right arm only.
3. Tell patient the above when he returns from having procedure for shunt placement.

M. Hill, R.N.

2-25-73 (1500) Nursing Progress Note
Problem #2—Reduced kidney function
Subjective data: Didn't mind procedure for it means can go home tomorrow.
Objective data: Pulse palpable at shunt site in left wrist. Patient demonstrated ability to test for shunt "buzz" c̄ fingers. No hand edema. No mention of future dialysis or transplant.
Assessment: Patient may not be ready to talk about dialysis and transplant and insufficient time ā discharge to adequately explore this c̄ him.
Plan: Continue observation of shunt per medical order.

Problem #2—Control of hypertension
   Subjective data: None.
   Objective data: Prescription obtained for patient. Medication schedule planned c̄ patient; recording system devised.
   Assessment: Feel patient understands and will correctly take and record medication.
   Plan: None.

                                                                    M. Hill, R.N.

2-26-73 (1200) Nursing Discharge Note
   This was the 1st General Hospital admission for John Roberts, a 30 year old single man from Springer, Florida admitted 2-19-73 for treatment of hypertension and evaluation of kidney function and discharged to home 2-26-73 to return for hemodialysis (schedule yet to be arranged) and future kidney transplant.

Problems	Noted	Resolved/Active
1. Control of hypertension	2-19-73	Active
2. Reduced kidney function	2-19-73	Active
A. Diet restriction	2-19-73	Resolved 2-23-73
B. Intake-output balance	2-19-73	Resolved 2-22-73
3. Blurred vision	2-19-73	Resolved 2-22-73
A. Dizziness	2-20-73	Resolved 2-21-73
4. Religion important to patient	2-19-73	Resolved 2-20-73

Problem #1—Control of hypertension
   Subjective data: None.
   Objective data: Patient's B.P. at medical objective of 90 mm. diastolic on prescribed dosage of Aldomet. Patient has prescription, medication schedule, and method for recording. Have asked patient to bring record c̄ him to first clinic visit 1 week from today at which time I will discuss procedure and any problems he might have had c̄ him.
   Assessment: Seems to understand medications, how to take, side effects and precautions he should take. Believe will take medication as ordered.
   *Plan:*None.

Problem #2—Reduced kidney function
   Subjective data: None.
   Objective data: Shunt in left wrist is working c̄ no swelling or bleeding observed. Patient demonstrated how to test shunt's working. Will be seeing local physician on 2-28-73 and to return to our clinic in 1 week. Has been told that he is in for a long work-up for kidney transplant and that his relatives will be worked up for compatibility. He may or may not be admitted to hospital again until June just before the transplant,

but he will be back to the clinic and dialysis unit. I felt that it was premature to talk about work up procedures and transplant except in very general terms.

Assessment: Knows how to care for shunt. Has demonstrated that he will follow instructions and seems to like to do what he can to participate in his care (such as recording own I and O, making sample menus). Will ask questions when he does not understand what is happening or what he is to do.

Plan: Will talk c̄ nurses in clinic and dialysis unit to explain that I have done little or no exploration c̄ patient concerning dialysis or transplant, but that it will need to be done as he moves through the kidney transplant program.

M. Hill, R.N.
General Hospital
Medical Unit
Phone: 635-3293

SECTION THREE

Appendices

APPENDIX 1: Clinical Nursing Tool

APPENDIX 2: Scientific Method

APPENDIX 3: Abbreviations

Appendix 1

CLINICAL NURSING TOOL

Part A. Nursing History: guide for the collection and organization of data.

    I. Vital statistics
   II. Patient's understanding of illness
  III. Some indications of the patient's expectations
  IV. Brief social and cultural history
   V. Significant data in terms of:
      A. Sleeping patterns
      B. Eliminating patterns
      C. Breathing
      D. Eating and drinking patterns
      E. Skin integrity
      F. Activity
      G. Recreation
      H. Interpersonal and communicative patterns
      I. Temperament
      J. Dependency and independency patterns
      K. Senses
      L. Menstrual patterns
  VI. Statement of that which makes the patient feel cared for (i.e., secure, comfortable, protected, safe).

Part B. Process of clinical thinking based on obtained data and appropriate parameters of knowledge.

    I. Numbered up-to-date problem list.
   II. Discussion of each problem, including identification of related factors which may enhance or inhibit the solving of the problem.
  III. Plan:
      A. The nursing care objectives in terms of patient behavior.

B. The intent to give information.

C. The intent to gather additional data.

IV. Implementation of the plan:

    A. The nursing orders by which the nursing care objectives are to be achieved.

    B. How information is to be given.

    C. How additional data is to be gathered.

V. Evaluation of nursing care through problem-related progress notes.

VI. Modification, addition and/or deletion of the plan in light of the patient's progress.

VII. Discharge, transfer, or expiration note.

Appendix 2

SCIENTIFIC METHOD

Definition:

A procedure for approaching a question, situation, person, or idea according to a definitely established, logical, and systematic plan.

Stages:

1. Collection of data.
2. Statement of the problem.

   The term problem is used to mean a question proposed for solution or consideration; anything required to be done. A problem is any condition or situation in which a patient requires help to maintain or regain a state of health, or to achieve a peaceful death. A problem may concern the patient, the patient's family, and/or the nurse. However, the problem must be based upon data obtained from the patient, the family and/or other members of the health team.
3. Analysis of the problem.

   This stage includes the study of existing knowledge. It necessitates consideration of all identifiable factors or phenomena contributing to the problem.
4. Selection of the phenomena to be studied.
5. Induction.

   The inductive stage includes the observation, description, and classification of the phenomena selected to be studied.
6. Statement of the relevant hypotheses.
7. Deduction.

   There are two parts to the deductive stage:
   A. Formulating postulates (assumptions or consequences) from each hypothesis.
   B. Testing each postulate by observation, study, and experiment.

If the hypothesis is found to be incorrect, another hypothesis must be chosen and the process of testing must be repeated.

8. Clarification of the relationship of the verified hypotheses to the initial problem.

9. Generalization to other situations.

When generalizing, one states how the information found through study of the problem can apply in other instances similar to the one studied.

Appendix 3

ABBREVIATIONS

ā — before
aa. — of each
a.c. — before meals
ab lib. — as desired
A.M. — morning
b.i.d. — twice each day
B.M. — bowel movement
B.P. — blood pressure
BR. — bathroom
BR.P. — bathroom privileges
c̄ — with
C. — Centigrade
cc. — cubic centimeter(s)
cm. — centimeter(s)
E.C.G. (also E.K.G.) — electrocardiogram
E.E.G. — electroencephalogram
fl. — fluid
gal. — gallon
Gm. — gram(s)
gr. — grain(s)
gtt. — drop(s)
H or hr. — hour
h.s. — hour of sleep
ht. — height
I.C.U. — Intensive Care Unit
I.M. — intramuscularly
I and O — intake and output
I.P.P.B. — intermittent positive pressure breathing

I.V. — intravenously; also used to refer to the intravenous infusion set-up.
Kg. — kilogram(s)
L. — liter(s)
lb. — pound(s)
mg. — milligram(s)
ml. — milliliter(s)
mm. — millimeter(s)
MOM — milk of magnesia
N/G — nasogastric
N.P.O. — nothing by mouth
O.O.B. — out of bed
O.D. — right eye
O.S. — left eye
O.T. — occupational therapy
O.U. — both eyes
oz. — ounce(s)
p̄ — after
p.c. — after meals
p.o. — by mouth
P.M. — afternoon
P.R.N. — whenever necessary
pt. — pint
Pt. — patient
P.T. — physical therapy
q. — every
q.d. — every day
q.h. — every hour
q.i.d. — four times daily

167

q.o.d. — every other day
qt. — quart
R.O.M. — range of motion
R.T. — radiotherapy or radiation therapy
Rx — treatment or therapy
s̄ — without
s.c. — subcutaneous
S.O.B. — shortness of breath

s̄s̄ — one half
stat. — at once
Tbsp. — tablespoon
t.i.d. — three times daily
T.P.R. — temperature, pulse, and respiration
V.S. — vital signs
wt. — weight

BIBLIOGRAPHY

Abdellah, Faye G.: "Criterion measures in nursing." *Nursing Research* X:21–26, 1961.
—— et al.: *Patient-Centered Approaches to Nursing*. The Macmillan Company, New York, 1964.
——, and Levine, Eugene: *Better Patient Care Through Nursing Research*. The Macmillan Company, New York, 1965.
"American Nurses' Association's first position on education for nursing." *American Journal of Nursing*, 65:106–111, 1965.
Arbuckle, Dugald S.: *Counseling: Philosophy, Theory, and Practice*. Allyn and Bacon, Inc., Boston, 1965.
Beland, Irene L.: *Clinical Nursing—Pathophysiological and Psychosocial Approaches*, second edition. The Macmillan Company, New York, 1970.
Benjamin, Alfred: *The Helping Interview*. Houghton Mifflin Company, Boston, 1969.
Beveridge, W. I. B.: *The Art of Scientific Investigation*, third edition. W. W. Norton and Company, Inc., New York, 1957.
Bingham, Walter Van Dyke, and Moore, Bruce Victor: *How to Interview*, fourth revised edition. Harper and Row, Publishers, New York, 1959.
Bjorn, John C., and Cross, Harold D.: *The Problem-Oriented Private Practice of Medicine*. Modern Hospital Press (McGraw-Hill Publications Company), Chicago, 1970.
Bloom, Benjamin S.: *Taxonomy of Educational Objectives: The Classification of Educational Goals, Handbook I: The Cognitive Domain*. David McKay Company, Inc., New York, 1956.
Bloom, Judith T., et al.: "Problem-oriented charting." *American Journal of Nursing*, 71:2144–2148, 1971.
Bower, Fay Louise: *The Process of Planning Nursing Care*. The C. V. Mosby Company, St. Louis, 1972.
Brammer, Lawrence M., and Shostrom, Everett L.: *Therapeutic Psychology: Fundamentals of Counseling and Psychotherapy*. Prentice-Hill, Inc., Englewood Cliffs, 1960.
Brodt, Dagmar E.: "Nursing care evaluation: Patient welfare parameters." Report of an investigation supported by United States Public Health Service Grant number NU-00170-01 from the Division of Nursing, Bureau of State Services, Community Health.
——, and Anderson, Ellen H.: "Validation of a patient welfare evaluation instrument." *Nursing Research* 16:167–169, 1967.
Chambers, Wilda: "Nursing diagnosis." *The American Journal of Nursing* 62:102–104, 1962.
Cohen, Sheldon: "Understanding and misunderstanding: What do you mean? How do you know?" *Insight*, Fall, 1966, pp. 1–13.
Cowan, Gregory, and McPherson, Elisabeth: *Plain English Please*. Random House, New York, 1966.
Dinsdale, Sidney M. et al.: "The problem-oriented medical record in rehabilitation." *Archives of Physical Medicine and Rehabilitation*, 51:488–492, 1970.

Durand, Mary, and Prince, Rosemary: "Nursing diagnosis: Process and decision." *Nursing Forum* V:50–64, 1966.

Durr, Carol A.: "Hands that help . . . But how?" *Nursing Forum* X:392–400, 1971.

Fenlason, Anne F.: *Essentials in Interviewing*. Harper and Row, Publishers, New York, 1952.

Field, Frances W.: "Communication between community nurse and physician." *Nursing Outlook* 19:722–725, 1971.

Foster, John, Jr.: *Science Writer's Guide*. Columbia University Press, New York, 1963.

Greenhill, Maurice H.: "Interviewing with a purpose." *American Journal of Nursing* 56:1259–1262, 1956.

Greenwood, Ernest: "The practice of science and the science of practice," in Bennis, W. C., Benne, K. D., and Chin, R. (Eds.): *Planning for Change*. Holt, Rinehart, and Winston, 1961.

Harmer, Bertha, and Henderson, Virginia; *Textbook of the Principles and Practice of Nursing*, Fifth edition. The Macmillan Company, New York, 1957.

Hays, Joyce Samhammer: "Analysis of nurse-patient communications." *Nursing Outlook* 14:32–35, 1966.

———, and Larson, Kenneth H.; *Interacting with Patients*. The Macmillan Company, New York, 1963.

Henderson, Virginia: *The Nature of Nursing: A Definition and Its Implications for Practice, Research, and Education*. The Macmillan Company, New York, 1966.

Herrmann, George R.: *Clinical Case-Taking*, fourth edition. The C. V. Mosby Company, St. Louis, 1949.

Hewitt, Helen E., and Pesznecker, Betty L.: "Blocks to communicating with patients." *American Journal of Nursing* 64:101–103, 1964.

Hurst, J. Willis: "Ten reasons why Lawrence Weed is right," (editorial). *The New England Journal of Medicine* 284:51–52, 1971.

——— "How to implement the Weed System: In order to improve patient care, education, and research by improving medical records." *Archives of Internal Medicine* 128:456–462, 1971.

———: "The Problem-Oriented Record and the Measurement of Excellence," *Archives of Internal Medicine*, 128:818–819, November, 1971.

———, and Walker, H. Kenneth (eds.): *The Problem-Oriented System*, MEDCOM, Inc., New York, 1957.

Kahn, Robert L., and Cannell, Charles F.: *The Dynamics of Interviewing*. John Wiley and Sons, Inc., New York, 1957.

Kelly, Nancy Cardinal: "Nursing care plans." *Nursing Outlook* 14:61–64, 1966.

Komorita, Nori I.: "Nursing diagnosis." *American Journal of Nursing* 63:83–86, 1963.

Mager, Robert F.: *Preparing Instructional Objectives*. Fearon Publishers, Inc., Palo Alto, 1962.

Marshall, Jon C., and Feeney, Sally: "Structured versus intuitive intake interview." *Nursing Research* 21:269–272, 1972.

Maslow, Abraham H.: "A Theory of Human Motivation." *Psychological Review* 50:370–396, 1943.

———: *Motivation and Personality*, Harper and Row, Publishers, New York, 1954.

———: *The Farther Reaches of Human Nature*. The Viking Press, New York, 1971.

McCain, R. Faye: "Nursing by assessment—not intuition." *American Journal of Nursing* 65:82–84, 1965.

Meadows, Lloyd, and Gass, Gertrude Zemon: "Problems of the novice interviewer." *American Journal of Nursing* 63:97–99, 1963.

Menzies, Isabel E. P.: *The Functioning of Social Systems as a Defense Against Anxiety*. Centre for Applied Social Research, The Tavistock Institute of Human Relations, Tavistock Centre, London, 1970.

Milhous, Raymond L.: "The problem-oriented medical record in rehabilitation management and training." *Archives of Physical Medicine and Rehabilitation* 53:182–185, 1972.

Miller, George E., et al: *Teaching and Learning in Medical School*. Harvard University Press, Cambridge, 1961.

Mosher, Frederic A., and Hornsby, Joan Rigney: "On asking questions," in *Studies in Cognitive Growth* (a Collaboration at the Center for Cognitive Studies), John Wiley and Sons, Inc., New York, 1966.

Mumford, Emily, and Skipper, James K.: *Sociology in Hospital Care.* Harper and Row, Publishers, New York, 1967.

Nightingale, Florence: *Notes on Nursing: What It Is and What It Is Not.* Harrison and Sons, London, 1859.

Northrop, F.S.C.: *The Logic of the Sciences and the Humanities.* The Macmillan Company, New York, 1947.

Orlando, Ida Jean: *The Dynamic Nurse-Patient Relationship,* G. P. Putnam's Sons, New York, 1961.

Peplau, Hildegard E.: *Interpersonal Relations in Nursing.* G. P. Putnam's Sons, New York, 1952.

———: "Talking with patients." *American Journal of Nursing* 60:964–966, 1960.

Phaneuf, Maria C.: *The Nursing Audit: Profile for Excellence.* Appleton-Century-Crofts, Educational Division/Meredith Corporation, New York, 1972.

Porterfield, John D.: "Joint Commission on Accreditation of Hospitals." *American Journal of Nursing* 71:70–73, 1971.

"The problem-oriented record as a basic tool in medical education, patient care, and clinical research," (editorial). *Annals of Clinical Research* 3:131–134, 1971.

Prosen, Harry: "Interviewing and understanding patients." *General Practitioners,* XXXV:95–98, 1967.

Richardson, Stephan A., Dohrenwend, Barbara Snell, and Klein, David: *Interviewing: Its Forms and Functions.* Basic Books, Inc., Publishers, New York, 1965.

Schwartz, Doris R.: "Toward more precise evaluation of patients' needs." *Nursing Outlook* 13:42–44, 1965.

Smith, Dorothy M.: "Myth and method in nursing practice." *American Journal of Nursing* 64:68–72, 1964.

———: "Nursing reformation," Unpublished Keynote Address delivered at the Florida Nurses' Association's Annual Convention, Hollywood, Florida, October 22, 1968.

———: "A clinical nursing tool." *American Journal of Nursing* 68:2384–2388, 1968.

———: "Is it too late?" *Nursing Clinics of North America,* W. B. Saunders Company, Philadelphia, 6:225–230, 1971.

———: "Writing of objectives as a nursing practice skill," *American Journal of Nursing* 71:319–320, 1971.

Smith, Henry Clay: *Sensitivity to People.* McGraw-Hill Book Company, New York, 1966.

Stevenson, Ian: *Medical History-Taking.* Harper and Row, Publishers, New York, 1960.

Travelbee, Joyce: *Interpersonal Aspects of Nursing.* F. A. Davis Company, Philadelphia, 1966.

Vanderzanden, James W., and Vanderzanden, Marion V.: "The interview—What questions should the nurse ask and how should she ask them?" *Nursing Outlook* 11:743–745, 1963.

Weed, Lawrence L., "Medical records, patient care, and medical education." *Irish Journal of Medical Science* 6:271–282, 1964.

——— "A new approach to medical teaching." *Medical Times* September, 1966, pp. 1030–1038.

———: "Medical records that guide and teach." *The New England Journal of Medicine* 278:593–600, 652–657; 1968.

——— "What physicians worry about: How to organize care of multiple-problem patients." *Modern Hospital* 110:90–94, 1968.

——— *Medical Records, Medical Education, and Patient Care,* The Press of Case Western Reserve University, Cleveland, Year Book Medical Publishers, Inc., Chicago, 1969.

——— "Quality Control and the Medical Record," *Archives of Internal Medicine* 127:101–105, January, 1971.

Weiss, Joseph J., and Yanez, Jose: "The problem oriented record: A new approach to total patient care." *Medical Times* 98:135–143, 1970.

Willard, Marian C.: "A matter of facts." *Nursing Outlook* 11:832–834, 1963.

Wilson, E. Bright, Jr.: *An Introduction to Scientific Research.* McGraw-Hill Book Company, Inc., New York, 1952.

Wooden, Howard E., and Smith, Dorothy M.: "Care programming and the nursing analysis." A Progress Report, Research Project NU00131, August 30, 1965.

Zimmerman, Donna Stielgis, and Gohrke, Carol: "The goal-directed nursing approach: It does work." *American Journal of Nursing* 70:306–310, 1970.

INDEX

173

174

175